The Bedside Dysmorphologist

The Bedside Dysmorphologist

Classic Clinical Signs in Human Malformation Syndromes
and Their Diagnostic Significance

William Reardon, M.D.

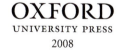

OXFORD
UNIVERSITY PRESS
2008

OXFORD
UNIVERSITY PRESS

Oxford University Press, Inc., publishes works that further
Oxford University's objective of excellence
in research, scholarship, and education.

Oxford   New York
Auckland   Cape Town   Dar es Salaam   Hong Kong   Karachi
Kuala Lumpur   Madrid   Melbourne   Mexico City   Nairobi
New Delhi   Shanghai   Taipei   Toronto

With offices in
Argentina   Austria   Brazil   Chile   Czech Republic   France   Greece
Guatemala   Hungary   Italy   Japan   Poland   Portugal   Singapore
South Korea   Switzerland   Thailand   Turkey   Ukraine   Vietnam

Copyright © 2008 by Oxford University Press, Inc.

Published by Oxford University Press, Inc.
198 Madison Avenue, New York, New York 10016

www.oup.com

Oxford is a registered trademark of Oxford University Press

Library of Congress Cataloging-in-Publication Data
Reardon, William, 1960–
The bedside dysmorphologist / William Reardon.
p. ; cm.
Includes bibliographical references.
ISBN 978-0-19-530045-1
1. Abnormalities, Human—Diagnosis—Handbooks, manuals, etc.
2. Physical diagnosis—Handbooks, manuals, etc.   I. Title.
[DNLM: 1. Abnormalities—diagnosis—Handbooks.
2. Pediatrics—Handbooks.   3. Child.   4. Infant.   WS 39 R288b 2007]
QM691.R43 2007
616'.043—dc22   2006028127

9 8 7 6 5 4

Printed in the United States of America
on acid-free paper

Preface

Although it has not always been so, dysmorphology is nowadays well served with several fine books on the subject. Many of the leading practitioners of our discipline have committed their wisdom and experience to the page to the great benefit of their colleagues and admirers all around the world, not to mention the incalculable service to countless patients. Consequently, there exist now several reputable and authoritative texts and computerized databases on the diagnostic approach to the dysmorphic child, on summarized published information relating to individual syndromes, on classic examples of known syndromes, and on various other aspects of dysmorphology practice. Notwithstanding these considerable aids, reaching a specific diagnosis in the dysmorphic individual remains, for most of us, a formidable barrier.

Embarking as a very junior trainee in clinical genetics almost 20 years ago, I often found myself confused as to what exactly constituted an abnormal clinical sign, so often the springboard to final diagnosis. The vivid admiration I harbored then for colleagues possessed of the clinical gifts and experience underlying the recognition of such signs still burns bright. Many of my early days in training were spent looking up articles in journals seeking that perfect demonstration of a seminal clinical sign as a means of clarifying my confused state of mind. This should not in any way reflect upon the mentoring offered to me, which could not have been bettered, but rather should reflect on my own inadequacies faced with the struggle to master the language, the literature, and the seemingly limitless variation in clinical subtlety with which human malformation syndromes are wont to clothe themselves.

Although mastery has proven elusive, experience has offered both compensation and concern—compensation in that I have now learned enough to accept that nobody has all the answers in dysmorphology, but concern that the exact same problems that I personally recollect as a youthful trainee are still cited by young colleagues undertaking training in clinical genetics—for example, "How can I be sure if the ears are low set?" "Is it significant if there are deep plantar creases?" "What should I be thinking of if the patient has micropenis?"

Experienced dysmorphologists will hear in these questions the panicky voice of inexperience, and their diagnostic insight is absolutely correct! However, other clinicians, and perhaps pediatricians above all others, will hear in these questions their own authentic voices, the concerns that bedevil their daily practices as they examine their patients, and wonder whether an individual has a dysmorphic sign suggestive of an underlying syndrome or not. It has surprised me that, in all the excellent dysmorphology books published over the last two decades, so little emphasis has been placed on assisting the nonspecialist, whether trainee geneticist, pediatrician, or other clinical colleague, to recognize dysmorphic signs and to understand their possible significance. It appears to me that the literature of clinical genetics and dysmorphology is now so sophisticated and well organized as to be quite daunting for most nonspecialists. Listening to pediatrician colleagues, I hear that the gulf between our specialty and our nongenetic colleagues can appear insurmountable, notwithstanding our shared interests in the diagnosis of and care for the malformed patient. This is the background to the concept of the book I wish to write—one that seeks to make the clinical signs of malformation and the reasoning process deriving from their observation less arcane than currently appears to be the case. For trainees in clinical genetics, there is an exigency to become comfortable with these concepts before progressing to a more advanced state of knowledge, while for nongeneticist colleagues, it is my hope that this book will answer some of the questions most frequently posed as to why genetic diagnoses may seem so inaccessible.

Acknowledgments

Is there truly such a phenomenon as a sole-author book? While I alone have written the words between these covers and provided the pictures, unless otherwise acknowledged, any work of this nature represents the synthesis of many years of example, training, influences, and practical support on the part of others. Indeed, as C.G. Jung would agree, this is merely if the conscious is to be acknowledged. Foremost among such mentors in my case were Robin Winter and Michael Baraitser, to whose wisdom and generosity I owe so much. The excellent photographs herein have virtually all been taken by Dave Cullen; those that are less than perfect are mine. Lisa Malone, my longstanding and loyal secretary, has responded to my many calls for assistance with patient details and organization. Nevan and Isolt Reardon have continually encouraged me by their interest in the undertaking. A succession of trainees, most memorably Mudaffer Al-Mudaffer, Ethel Ryan, and Nichola Concannon, have voiced their concerns at possible clinical signs overlooked or misinterpreted and, in so doing, have reminded me of another, younger, self and have helped me to view the clinical dysmorphic examination through the prism of inexperience. For their candor and self-critical faculties, I am grateful. Jeff House and his successor at Oxford University Press, Bill Lamsback, both showed great enthusiasm for this book and have been unfailingly encouraging from initial idea to finished product. When short of a good clinical photograph to illuminate a specific point, I have been fortunate to be able to call on the support of clinical colleagues, among whom my friend, Ian Young, has been especially supportive. Finally, I must thank the many parents in my practice who consented to the inclusion of clinical photographs of their child.

Contents

Chapter 1 The Skull

Chapter 2 The Face

Chapter 3 The Eye and Related Structures

Chapter 4 The Ear

Chapter 5 The Mouth and Oral Cavity

Chapter 6 The Neck

Chapter 7 The Chest

Chapter 8 The Abdomen and Perineum

Chapter 9 The Hands

Chapter 10 The Feet

Chapter 11 The Limbs

Chapter 12 The Nails, Hair, and Skin

The Bedside Dysmorphologist

Chapter 1 The Skull

1.1 Plagiocephaly

Recognizing the Sign Plagiocephaly signifies asymmetry of the skull. It may involve the front or back of the skull. Most cases of posterior plagiocephaly simply reflect the position adopted by the infant in sleep and represent a classic example of a deformation. By contrast, anterior plagiocephaly is more frequently due to an underlying coronal suture synostosis. Surgical assessment and intervention may be necessary.

Establishing a Differential Diagnosis A diagnosis of anterior plagiocephaly poses two essential questions of the clinician: Is there an underlying syndrome and is there **craniosynostosis**?

Take a brief family history and observe the parents. Ask specifically whether anybody has had cranial surgery. Remember that within families, segregating dominant craniosynostosis individuals usually consider themselves entirely unremarkable and may be unaware of clinical features considered dysmorphic in a hospital setting. In examining the baby, important considerations to remember are whether the sutures of the skull actually *feel* synostotic. Generally in a plagiocephalic infant, if there is synostosis, it is confined to a single coronal suture, but it is worth palpating all sutures, especially the sagittal. The eyebrows and palpebral fissures will often show asymmetry in a unilateral coronal synostosis. Examine the thumbs and halluces. Wide halluces may suggest **Saethre-Chotzen syndrome** or synostosis due to pro250arg mutation of the *FGFR3* gene. Incomplete skin syndactyly between the digits and prominence of the crus helicis of the ears are good clinical signs for Saethre-Chotzen syndrome. Look at the skin for acanthosis nigricans, associated with a specific form of **Crouzon syndrome** and especially seen in the axillae and neck. Examine the genitalia, especially in females. Any suggestion of clitoromegaly may be the prompt to **Antley-Bixler syndrome** and, in such circumstances, the joints should be examined, as joint fusion or limitation will substantiate this likely diagnosis.

Investigations to Consider Skull x-rays will confirm or refute sutural synostosis. A karyotype may be valuable, especially in a dysmorphic child with normal parents. If a specific syndrome is suggested by the clinical features, mutation analysis of the *FGFR* gene family or other relevant loci may be warranted. Most clinically identifiable syndromic synostoses are single gene related and have normal chromosomes. If Antley-Bixler syndrome is suspected from large joint limitation/fusion or if there are concerns about genital development, a detailed assessment of the infant's steroid hormone status is indicated.

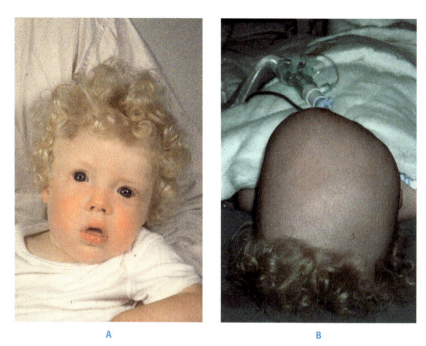

A   B

Figure 1.1A and B A right-sided plagiocephaly, caused by isolated coronal suture fusion, is shown. There is orbital asymmetry, the right eyebrow is distorted, and there is flattening of the right temporoparietal region. The preoperative photograph from above shows the frontal asymmetry more clearly.

1.2 Metopic Ridge

Recognizing the Sign The metopic suture is in the vertical plane in the midline of the forehead. Prominence of the metopic ridge is a normal, non-pathologic feature in more than 10% of children. However, it is also a non-specific feature seen in some dysmorphic disorders and, therefore, is not to be dismissed. Viewed from above, the anterior skull takes on a triangular appearance (trigonocephaly). From the front, the eyes may appear to be close together. An alternative descriptive term sometimes used is "keel-shaped skull." Most cases are not related to synostosis.

Establishing a Differential Diagnosis Diagnostic considerations associated with this sign and that merit directed history taking and examination are relatively limited. About 5% of cases of trigonocephaly with synostosis will have a positive family history of craniosynostosis, usually trigonocephalic. Some 20% of nonfamilial cases are associated with other malformations, often non-specific. Particular attention should be paid to a history of **sodium valproate exposure in pregnancy**, metopic ridging being a cardinal feature of the resultant malformation pattern. Poor growth and coarse features, often with lip fullness, should lead to evaluation for I-cell disease (mucolipidosis type II), particularly if gingival thickening or hepatosplenomegaly is observed. Facial hemangioma, particularly over the glabellar region, is an excellent clue to the diagnosis of **Oberklaid-Danks syndrome**. Other diagnostically valuable clinical signs in this condition are hypertelorism, cleft or deeply ridged palate, and abnormal wrist position, often with camptodactyly. Iris coloboma may signify an underlying diagnosis of **Baraitser-Winter syndrome**.

Investigations to Consider Radiologic examination may be necessary to exclude metopic suture synostosis. Basic karyotype is valuable, many chromosomal abnormalities being associated with trigonocephaly. The most common of these is **Jacobsen syndrome**, chromosome 11q deletion. Chromosome 9p deletion is also over-represented in trigonocephalic presentations, and it is worth drawing the particular attention of the cytogenetic laboratory to chromosomes 9 and 11 in the trigonocephalic presentation. As with any chromosomal deletion, a formal examination for other malformations, such as cardiac, should be undertaken. Vacuolated lymphocytes or cytoplasmic inclusions on fibroblast microscopy will be consistent with I-cell disease. Notwithstanding their association with craniosynostosis, *FGFR* gene mutations are very uncommon in trigonocephaly and rarely warranted. Magnetic resonance imaging (MRI) scan for frontal pachygyria or other evidence of neuronal migration defect will support a clinical suspicion of Baraitser-Winter syndrome.

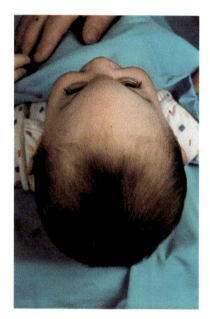

Figure 1.2A Trigonocephaly as a result of metopic sutural synostosis is demonstrated.

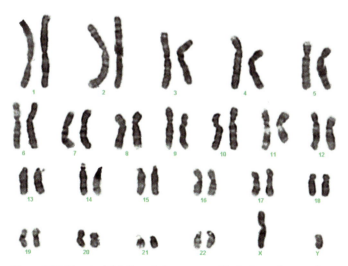

Figure 1.2B Terminal deletion of chromosome 11q is shown from a trigonocephalic, developmentally delayed child.

1.3 Scalp Defects

Recognizing the Sign The term is self-explanatory, the real issue being to determine whether or not it has a wider diagnostic significance. Note that some defects are not confined to the scalp and may involve skull vault bony deficiencies, and severe bleeding events have been reported from the site of the defect. Even in adult life, the healed scalp defect is usually hairless. Most scalp defects are benign and do not signify intracranial pathology or an associated syndromic diagnosis.

Establishing a Differential Diagnosis Benign isolated scalp defects may be familial, so take a family history and examine the affected child's parents. Specific inquiry of antenatal events may reveal **maternal ingestion of aspirin**. The clinical examination should direct specific attention to the skin for possible areas of aplasia cutis, which will suggest the condition of **aplasia cutis congenita**. Examine the hands and feet for signs of transverse limb defects, often subtle, which may signify **Adams-Oliver syndrome**. In that event, the heart merits careful evaluation, there being as association with congenital heart disease. Do not dismiss ring-like skin folds of a digit or limb, resembling amniotic bands, as these are well reported in Adams-Oliver syndrome. Assess the nipples for absence or hypoplasia and observe the external ears for thickening, overfolding of helices and absence of the tragus, any of which signs should prompt a diagnosis of **Finlay-Marks syndrome**, another autosomal dominant condition. Partial syndactyly of the fingers or toes would also be consistent with this diagnosis. The presence of epibulbar dermoids is diagnostically significant, prompting the closer examination of the skin for pigmentary abnormalities. Some children with epibulbar dermoids and scalp defects have developed giant cell granulomas. The pattern of hair growth, especially in the presence of a frontal upsweep, is a clue to **Johanson-Blizzard syndrome**. A history of failure to thrive and the observation of a small nose, specifically with hypoplastic alae nasi, would further support this autosomal recessive diagnosis as the reason for the scalp defect.

Investigations to Consider Do a cardiac assessment if the signs suggest Adams-Oliver syndrome. Karyotype is indicated in sporadic cases, and chromosomal abnormalities of trisomy 13 and deletion 4p are especially common. Audiologic assessment for deafness is indicated in Johanson-Blizzard cases, as are thyroid function measures and assessment for pancreatic insufficiency. Longitudinal clinical follow-up of cases with epibulbar dermoids is needed lest this be a cancer predisposition condition, evidence for which is currently suggestive but inconclusive.

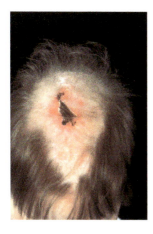

Figure 1.3A Healing scalp defect with surrounding hairless area is shown in a 3-year-old girl with aplasia cutis congenita.

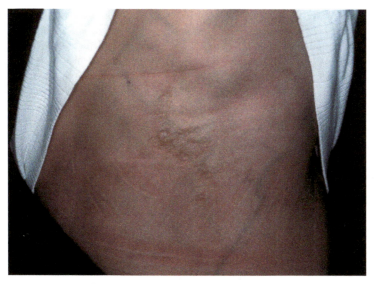

Figure 1.3B Localized region of aplasia cutis congenita in the mother of the child shown in Figure 1.3A.

1.4   Macrocephaly

Recognizing the Sign The sign itself is not difficult; rather, it's a question of definition. Its identification prompts concerns with respect to likely significance for brain development. History, examination, and investigation combine to assess this possible impact.

Establishing a Differential Diagnosis History and parental examination may offer evidence for a familial characteristic. Examination should assess body proportions, lest there is an underlying skeletal dysplasia, macrocephaly being a common finding in **hypochondroplasia** and many other similar disorders. Noteworthy frontal bossing and large chin are clues to **Sotos syndrome;** patients with this condition often have rather ruddy cheeks, in addition to developmental delay. Limb or trunk asymmetry may suggest **Proteus** or **Klippel-Trenaunay-Weber syndromes**. Polydactyly is important, possibly suggesting **Greig syndrome**, especially if there is parental macrocephaly. A parental history of surgical resection of polydactyly may be invaluable in securing this diagnosis. Although not invariable, the polydactyly of Greig syndrome is most commonly postaxial in the hands and preaxial in the feet. The skin may offer etiologic clues—facial hemangioma, especially of the upper lip, suggesting **macrocephaly-cutis marmorata telangiectasia congenita syndrome**, often with associated limb asymmetry and/or polydactyly. Verrucous lesions and/or lipomata raise concerns with respect to possible Proteus syndrome. The cutaneous signs of Cowden spectrum and Proteus syndromes overlap. Examine the glans penis for macules, seen in the **Bannayan-Zonana syndrome** form of the Cowden syndrome spectrum. Similarly, mucocutaneous papules, especially around the mouth and anus, involving hair follicles are good clues to **Cowden syndrome**. Be aware that these may not present until the second decade. The presence of café-au-lait patches should prompt a search for other clues to **neurofibromatosis type 1**, while accessory nipples may signal **Simpson-Golabi-Behmel syndrome**. Additional evidence for the latter might be gleaned from small nails on the index fingers, a deep midline groove on the tongue, or a history of diaphragmatic hernia. Look for hepatosplenomegaly, general coarseness, and gingival thickening as possible clues to a metabolic cause.

Investigations to Consider Skeletal radiology is indicated if a dysplasia is thought likely and bone age is indicated if Sotos syndrome is suspected. Organic acids for glutaric aciduria, mucopolysaccharide screen, and very-long-chain fatty acids may be indicated by concerns for a biochemical disorder. Basic karyotype will have a low yield but fragile X DNA evaluation should not be overlooked in the absence of clinical signs of other etiologies. A Dandy-Walker malformation on brain scan should prompt consideration of Meckel and Bardet-Biedl syndromes, while ventriculomegaly and thinning of the corpus callosum are known in several conditions such as Sotos and Greig syndromes.

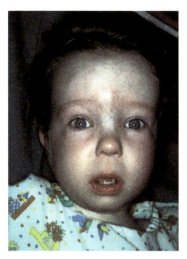

Figure 1.4A This macrocephalic patient has no specific diagnostic clinical features, as is often the case, but the macrocephaly is caused by a mutation of the *PTEN* gene, indicating the underlying diagnosis of the Cowden syndrome spectrum. The occipitofrontal head circumference (OFC) is 4 cm above the 97th percentile for age at 4 years.

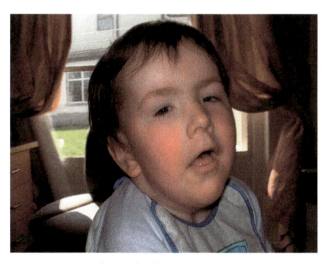

Figure 1.4B A typical example of Sotos syndrome is shown. Note the macrocephaly, prominent chin, and ruddy cheeks, often observed in Sotos syndrome patients.

1.5 Microcephaly

Recognizing the Sign Microcephaly is another easy sign to determine by definition, but is so very important prognostically and so diagnostically bewildering as to be something of a clinician's nightmare.

Establishing a Differential Diagnosis Several "pure" microcephaly conditions are autosomal recessive, and the history must address this possibility by specifically seeking evidence for consanguinity. Likewise, antenatal exposure to infection or teratogenic agents needs to be eliminated. Assess whether the microcephaly is genuine or reflective of a general growth disturbance. Organomegaly, macroglossia, gingival hyperplasia, or unusual smell may suggest a biochemical disorder as the basic underlying pathology. Specific dysmorphic signs may pinpoint a known syndrome—bitemporal narrowing and 2/3 toe syndactyly suggest **Smith-Lemli-Opitz syndrome**, while more extensive syndactyly of toes and fingers is consistent with **Filippi syndrome**. Thumb hypoplasia prompts thoughts of **Fanconi syndrome,** and a skin examination for pigmented areas should follow. Short first metacarpals and synophrys suggest **de Lange syndrome**, while telangiectasia may be the clue to **Bloom syndrome**. Examine the eyes—blood vessels visible in the lateral canthus should lead to examination of the eyebrows for sparse areas or interruption, characteristics of **Kabuki syndrome**. Deep-set eyes should provoke inquiry about sun sensitivity and photophobia, often the clues to **Cockayne syndrome**. Small ears suggest **Meier-Gorlin syndrome**, confirmed by absent patellae, while large ears should prompt evaluation of calcium, often low in **Richardson-Kirk syndrome**. Inversion of the nipples and unusual fat distribution are clues to the **carbohydrate-deficient glycoprotein** (CDG) disorders.

Investigations to Consider Investigation will be led by the conclusions of history and examination. A basic karyotype is valuable, nowadays often supplemented by specific fluorescence in situ hybridization (FISH) analysis or DNA mutation search, depending on the clinical signs. Premature chromosome condensation is an important observation, being specific to pure autosomal recessive microcephaly type 1 associated with mutation at the *MCPH1* locus on chromosome 8. Sister chromatid exchange is indicated in the presence of telangiectasis, while diepoxybutane challenge is warranted if Fanconi syndrome is considered likely. Basic blood parameters may show pancytopenia in the latter. Disordered blood indices are also suggestive of CDG disorders, for which conditions transferrin isoelectric focusing is the investigation of choice. Increased levels of 7-dehydrocholesterol are characteristic of Smith-Lemli-Opitz syndrome. Neuroradiology may give a descriptive diagnosis of a brain malformation disorder, many of which are due to single gene mutation, and the relevant search at the specific locus may be repaid with a confirmatory diagnosis.

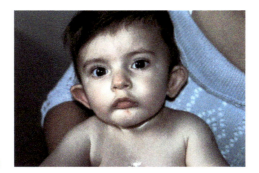

A

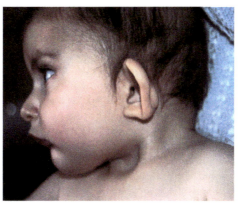

B

Figure 1.5A and B The clinical clue to the underlying diagnosis of Richardson-Kirk syndrome, an autosomal recessive disorder, in this microcephalic child lies in the observation of low-set, prominent ears. Note also the rather deep-set eyes. Serum calcium was low in the neonatal period.

1.6 Frontal Hairline Variants—High Hairline and Frontal Upsweep

Recognizing the Sign One does not measure the position of the frontal hairline, but rather forms an impression of its relative position in terms of other landmarks, such as the orbit. A wide degree of interindividual variation is normal and, even if noticeably high, there is not a consistent relationship with pathologic syndromes. If the hairline is "high," the temporoparietal skin is more visible than usual. In general, the hair lies forward at the frontal hairline, and a reversal of this, with the hair swept backward, is frontal upsweep, also know as cowlick.

Establishing a Differential Diagnosis High hairline may be familial, especially in **tricho-rhino-phalangeal (TRP) syndrome**, which is inherited in an autosomal dominant manner. Clinical signs of particular diagnostic value to assess in the parents and child if this diagnosis is being considered are a bulbous nose and wide middle phalanges of the fingers, which may also show ulnar deviation. Syndromes involving **craniosynostosis** can distort the frontal hairline, so be aware of skull shape and familial appearances in assessing frontal hairline in a baby. Persisting temporal absence of hair in an older child should prompt thoughts of **Pallister-Killian syndrome**, especially if developmental delay is likely. In the older child with short stature and apparent failure to thrive, a high hairline may be the clue to **Mulibrey nanism**, in which case relative macrocephaly is common.

Frontal upsweep is unmistakable, being a normal variant in most instances. However, it is a characteristic finding in **Johanson-Blizzard syndrome**, in which condition the very pinched nose with hypoplastic alae nasi will secure the diagnosis. There is often an associated scalp defect and a range of cardiac malformations described make cardiac consultation advisable if this diagnosis is being considered. In the presence of severe developmental delay in a male child with noteworthy frontal upsweep, consider the likelihood of **X-linked α-thalassemia and mental retardation** (ATRX). The family history may offer further encouragement to pursue this possible diagnosis. Upsweep is also seen in **Rubinstein-Taybi syndrome** (R-TS), most such cases showing the characteristic wide, deviated thumbs. **FG syndrome** patients whose main problems are constipation and developmental delay may often show a frontal upsweep.

Investigations to Consider Karyotype for chromosome 8q deletion is valuable in TRP syndrome, while skin chromosome analysis may be necessary to unmask the tetrasomy 12p in Pallister-Killian syndrome, chromosomes usually being normal in lymphocytes. Retinal pigment dots and fibrous dysplasia of the long bones, particularly the fibula, would support Mulibrey nanism. Diagnostic concerns for ATRX should prompt a search for HbH inclusion bodies using freshly constituted brilliant cresyl blue stain. Mutation analysis is available for ATRX and R-T syndromes.

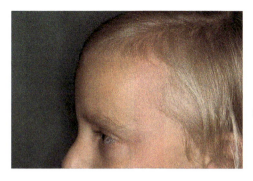

Figure 1.6A High hairline is demonstrated in a typical case of tricho-rhino-phalangeal syndrome. Observe how sparse the hair is frontally.

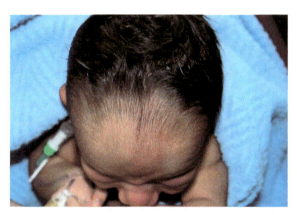

Figure 1.6B Frontal up-sweep, in this instance in a patient with Johanson-Blizzard syndrome.

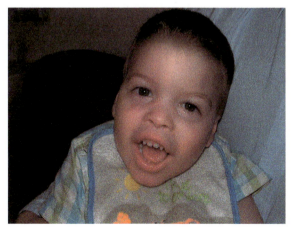

Figure 1.6 C A typical cowlick of the anterior hairline is shown in this patient with X-linked α-thalassemia mental retardation syndrome.

1.7 Frontal Hairline Variants—Low Hairline and Widow's Peak

Recognizing the Sign In fetal life, the extension of scalp hair growth onto the face is suppressed by circular regions around the eyes and ears, thus forming the normal scalp anterior margin. Eyelashes and eyebrows are exempt from this regulation. Widow's peak is the term used to describe a midline prominence of the frontal hairline, while a low frontal hairline refers to the downward extension of hair onto the temple toward the lateral eyebrow.

Establishing a Differential Diagnosis Widow's peak is a normal observation in most instances, often the consequence of mild hypertelorism, due to lateral shift of the hair growth suppression zones around the orbit. Consequently, a slight tongue of hair extends forward in the midline. If present, there are specific features to now look out for—a nasal tip groove suggests a diagnosis of **frontonasal dysplasia**, while the presence of craniosynostosis, often unilateral coronal fusion, will signify a diagnosis of **craniofrontonasal dysplasia** (CFND). Longitudinal ridges along the nails, which often split in this plane, are characteristic findings in CFND and diagnostically valuable is demarcating this condition from other disorders with widow's peak. Pigmentary irregularities of the iris or skin may be the clues to **Waardenburg syndrome**, usually type I, in which associated widow's peak is often observed. A family history of early hair greying, dying of specific areas of grey hair, and deafness will support this diagnosis. A shawl configuration to the scrotum in a boy with widow's peak could well be the clue to a diagnosis of **Aarskog syndrome**, especially if he is of short stature.

A low frontal hairline should draw the clinician's attention to the eyes, as it is an almost invariable presence in **Fraser syndrome**. Interruption to the margin of the alae nasi in the form of a notch, dysplastic ears, and skin syndactyly of the fingers would further support this autosomal recessive diagnostic conclusion, as would genital anomalies. Hairline distortion may reflect underlying **craniosynostosis**, so attention to head shape in the individual and family is warranted. Check specifically for an antenatal history of **phenytoin exposure**, the temporal extension of hair being documented. A cheekward extension of a tongue-like projection of hair is common in **Treacher Collins syndrome**, so it is worth looking for pinna abnormalities, lower eyelid colobomata, and maxillary hypoplasia.

Investigations to Consider Skull radiology is indicated if craniosynostosis is suspected. In Fraser syndrome, consider ophthalmologic evaluation, renal ultrasound, brain neuroimaging, and, possibly, DNA studies. Computed tomography (CT) scan of the petrous temporal bone in Treacher Collins should be obtained to establish the degree of ossicular malformation.

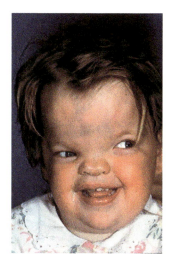 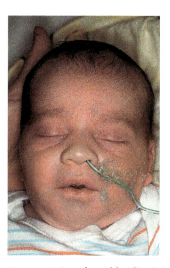

Figure 1.7A Widow's peak is demonstrated in a patient with craniofrontonasal dysplasia. Note also the hypertelorism, narrow palpebral fissures, and the bifid nasal tip.

Figure 1.7B Low frontal hairline is demonstrated. Note also the significant infraorbital skin groove, betraying the underlying diagnosis of Schinzel-Gideon syndrome in this patient.

1.8 Low Posterior Hairline

Recognizing the Sign Scalp hair extending downward onto the neck is thought to reflect prenatal nuchal edema. Unsurprisingly then, posterior hairline anomalies often accompany excess skin, referred to as neck webbing, but may equally represent the clinical clue to structural malformations of the cervical vertebrae. The term "trident hairline" is sometimes used, meaning three-pronged appearance, and simply reflects a particular pattern of low posterior hairline, wherein an M-shaped margin to the hairline is discerned.

Establishing a Differential Diagnosis Once sure that the posterior hairline is indeed low, assess the neck for redundant skin. In a neonate, the additional presence of puffy feet is suggestive of lymphoedema and a likely diagnosis of **Turner syndrome**. Examine the heart and check for brachiofemoral delay, specifically in view of the common association between Turner syndrome and coarctation of the aorta. Significant clinical overlap exists with **Noonan syndrome**, in which condition a history of a parent having had a congenital heart lesion may be elicited or other clinically supportive evidence, such as ptosis, adduced. Parental auscultation for unsuspected cardiac murmur is often valuable. Beware of bleeding defects in Noonan cases; a history of prolonged gum bleeding following tooth extraction in the parent of a child with low posterior hairline can alert the astute clinician to this diagnosis. The emergence of café-au-lait skin patches in the preschool child is significant and probably indicative of Noonan-NF syndrome, a variant of **neurofibromatosis type 1,** which therefore puts the child at risk for optic glioma, renal artery stenosis, pheochromocytoma, and other complications attendant upon NF1. Segmentation defects of the cervical spine should be considered in patients with low posterior hairline. Confirmation of cervical vertebral fusion, **Klippel-Feil syndrome**, should be followed by investigation of the renal tract, agenesis, hypoplasia, and ureteric duplication being common associations. Vaginal atresia and/or absent uterus are frequent in females with cervical vertebral fusions, while bilateral absence of the vas deferens, cryptorchidism, and similar renal anomalies represent the typical male profile.

Investigations to Consider Formal cardiac evaluation is indicated if Turner syndrome or Noonan syndrome is considered. This may extend to other family members in Noonan syndrome. Coagulation assessment is useful in Noonan syndrome, particularly if minor surgical procedures are being contemplated outside of a hospital environment. Karyotype will be definitive in Turner syndrome. Neck x-ray to assess cervical vertebrae is valuable in non-Turner, non-Noonan cases. Ultrasonic evaluation of the genitourinary tract structures is important in Klippel-Feil and related syndromes.

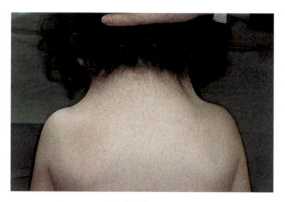

Figure 1.8 Low posterior hairline is associated with very noteworthy neck webbing in this 3-year-old girl with Noonan syndrome who had first come to attention when an antenatal scan at 26 weeks' gestation showed hydrops fetalis.

1.9 Anencephaly

Recognizing the Sign Conventional wisdom represents the primary event in anencephaly as failure of closure of the anterior neural groove. In consequence, forebrain development is incomplete with calvarial defects and possible malformations of the face and its structures. The spectrum of resultant clinical phenotypes represents a sequence of disordered embryologic and fetal developmental processes arising from this single primary event. It follows that a natural degree of clinical variability is to be anticipated between cases. Most cases represent variants of the spina bifida disease spectrum and are not associated with specific recognizable single gene syndromes or recurrence risks attendant upon single gene disorders. The purpose of clinical examination is to identify cases that represent clinical presentation of syndromes, many of them of autosomal recessive inheritance, whose recognition will have profound consequences for genetic counseling.

Establishing a Differential Diagnosis A range of **environmental** agents, alcohol, valproate, and rubella are all confirmed causes of meningocele, though less convincingly of anencephaly. This association will not be substantiated without dutiful antenatal history taking in future cases! Specifically examine the hands and feet. Small thumbs or absent thumbs lead to evaluation of the radii. The forearms may be shortened clinically and radiologic radial malformations identified. Such observations will be consistent with a likely diagnosis of the **XK aprosencephaly syndrome**. Check for anal atresia or stenosis, which will help secure the diagnosis, if present. Likewise, hand and foot malformations attend **acrocallosal syndrome**, the "classical" pattern being preaxial polydactyly of the feet with or without postaxial polydactyly of the hands. This pattern is not absolute but emphasizes the diagnostic value of well-documented examination. **Meckel-Gruber syndrome** more typically presents a posterior encephalocele but anencephalic presentation is well described. The polydactyly is typically postaxial, but the most consistent clinical finding, and therefore that of greatest diagnostic value, is renal and hepatic cysts. Documentation of cysts will afford distinction from **hydrolethalus syndrome** in which preaxial and/or postaxial polydactyly with encephalocele or anencephaly are typical features, but often this diagnosis is signaled by the antenatal history of polyhydramnios.

Investigations to Consider Radiology of limb malformations, if present, and autopsy examination of infants with clinical features that prompt concerns about a syndromic presentation of anencephaly are the most important investigative considerations.

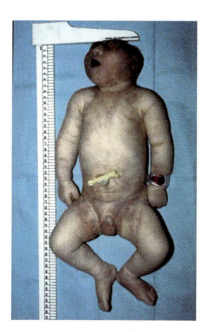

Figure 1.9 A typical example of anencephaly is shown. (Courtesy of Dr. Peter Kelehan.)

Chapter 2 The Face

2.1 Hypertelorism

Recognizing the Sign This term refers to widely spaced eyes and, by definition, the interpupillary distance is increased. A clinical impression of hypertelorism can be created by epicanthic folds, by a depressed nasal bridge, or by telecanthus, in which the inner canthus is displaced laterally, the inner canthus being the meeting point of the upper and lower eyelids on the medial side of the eye. A useful clinical guide is to assess whether an imaginary vertical line through the lacrimal punctum actually overlaps the iris. Should this be the case, then there is telecanthus. Thus, one's first clinical impression of hypertelorism needs to be more carefully assessed for possible confounding factors. Once satisfied that the patient does indeed manifest hypertelorism, the purpose of further examination is to evaluate the likely significance of this confirmed clinical sign.

Establishing a Differential Diagnosis A mild degree of hypertelorism, often with associated widow's peak, may be familial and benign. In terms of syndromic associations, the presence of a vertical groove of the nasal tip suggests the diagnosis of **frontonasal dysplasia**, while craniosynostosis and a nasal tip groove are consistent with **craniofrontonasal dysplasia**. Hoarseness of the voice should prompt questioning with respect to stridor, a history of neonatal feeding difficulty, or aspiration. These represent possible pointers to an underlying laryngeal cleft; and cause the clinician to examine for hypospadias—these being the cardinal features of **Opitz G syndrome**. Being an X-linked disorder, asymptomatic mothers may show mild clinical features. In the context of significant developmental delay in a male and increasing facial coarseness, best seen on serial photographs, with gathering prominence of the lips, thoughts of **Coffin-Lowry syndrome** would be justified. Many early cases of **α-thalassemia mental retardation syndrome** of the X-linked type (ATRX) were confused with Coffin-Lowry syndrome, the clinical features being very similar. Both are X-linked and may show mild features in carriers. The digits of Coffin-Lowry syndrome are often tapering and many geneticists point to the frequent observation of an accessory transverse hypothenar crease (Figure 9.9). In cases of mild developmental delay, especially if associated with short stature, the hypertelorism may be associated with **Aarskog syndrome**. Confirm clinically by observing the digits for brachydactyly, often with mild skin syndactyly; the scrotum will generally have a shawl configuration.

Investigations to Consider DNA mutation analysis is indicated for ATRX and Coffin-Lowry syndromes. HbH inclusion bodies on staining with freshly constituted brilliant cresyl blue is a good screening measure for ATRX and identifies 90% of cases. Skeletal survey in Aarskog syndrome often shows multiple epiphyseal dysplasia of mild degree.

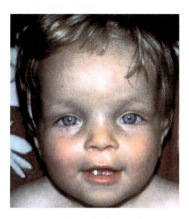

Figure 2.1A Note the hypertelorism in this patient with Aarskog syndrome. It is worth noting the wide philtrum. Contrast with the telecanthus of **Figure 2.1B**, where the inner canthus is laterally displaced, giving an impression of wide-spaced eyes.

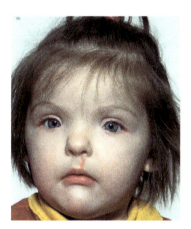

Figure 2.1B Note the medially flared eyebrows and synophrys, in addition to telecanthus, in this patient who has Waardenburg syndrome.

2.2 Hypotelorism

Recognizing the Sign By definition, the interpupillary distance is reduced. The clinical impression of hypotelorism should lead the experienced clinician to examine the patient for other clinical signs consonant with this feature and that may enhance the likelihood of identifying specific syndromes known to be associated with hypotelorism.

Establishing a Differential Diagnosis Metopic suture fusion, resulting in trigonocephaly, causes hypotelorism (1.2). Likewise, hypotelorism may be seen in nonspecific clinical situations such as **chromosomal trisomies and deletion** syndromes, which, by their nature, are of widely varying phenotype. Cyclopia, a single centrally placed eye, represents an extreme form of hypotelorism, and it is not surprising that varying degrees of hypotelorism are seen in **holoprosencephaly**, in which condition incomplete development of the frontal lobes of the brain is often associated with developmental failure of the olfactory tracts. Many of these children do not survive the neonatal period, but careful clinical examination of other family members may show clinical clues, in particular a single central incisor or anosmia. In association with 2/3 syndactyly of the toes, the autosomal recessive condition of **Smith-Lemli-Opitz syndrome** is an important differential diagnosis to investigate. Olfactory tract maldevelopment, resulting in anosmia, is also a feature of **Kallmann syndrome**, mostly an X-linked disorder and with associated clinical findings of cleft palate or uvula, mirror movements, and micropenis or failure of pubertal development, which is often the presenting feature. Renal agenesis is also associated. In the presence of skin syndactyly, particularly of fingers 3/4/5, think of **oculo-dento-digital syndrome** and seek a history of premature tooth decay. It is also worth examining for signs of spasticity, as white matter changes on magnetic resonance imaging (MRI) are well described, and asking if others in the family have needed digital surgery—the condition is autosomal dominant. In **Hallermann-Streiff syndrome**, the face is dominated by the narrow, prominent nose, but a high forehead, hypotelorism, and small chin will all support the likely diagnosis, as will cataracts.

Investigations to Consider Some 40% of holoprosencephaly cases have a chromosomal abnormality, most commonly trisomy 13. Mutations at six loci have been demonstrated on DNA analysis. 7-Dehydrocholesterol levels are indicated in suspected Smith-Lemli-Opitz syndrome, elevation thereof being diagnostic of this autosomal recessive condition. Xp chromosome deletion by fluorescence in situ hybridization (FISH) analysis or, if normal, mutation analysis of *KALL1* and *FGFR1* genes is indicated for likely cases of Kallmann syndrome.

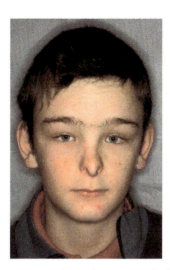

Figure 2.2A Note the narrow palpebral fissures in this boy with oculo-dento-digital syndrome. The inner canthi are slightly displaced, which ameliorates the impression of hypotelorism, but the interpupillary distance is reduced. Other important features to observe in this patient are synophrys and the hypoplastic alae nasi, which gives the nares a somewhat anteverted appearance (see 2.4 and 2.5).

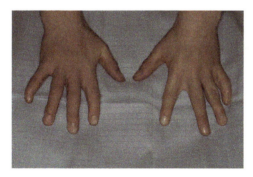

Figure 2.2B The hands of the patient in Figure 2.2A are demonstrated postsurgery for 3/4/5 syndactyly.

2.3 Abnormal Nasal Bridge

Recognizing the Sign The nasal bridge refers to the bony element of the nose between the orbits. The evaluation of this structure for dysmorphic signs is complicated by the range of normal variation in the population, shared familial traits, and age-related phenomena, specifically the observation that depression of the nasal bridge is the norm in infancy. Unsurprisingly then, a clinical impression of raised or depressed nasal bridge needs to be substantiated by other evidence if it is to enjoy diagnostic significance.

Establishing a Differential Diagnosis Widening of the nasal bridge is usual in hypertelorism, for which reason assessment of the nasal tip, the skin, general facial appearance, and height remain relevant (2.1). Nasal bridge widening is characteristic of **Waardenburg syndrome,** for which reason the clinician should evaluate the irides for heterochromia and eyelashes and hair for hypopigmented areas, in addition to querying the use of hair coloring products, a comment which equally applies to parents of an affected child. Observe for hearing or speech difficulties. A high nasal bridge, particularly in the context of developmental delay and truncal obesity, is characteristic of **Cohen syndrome** (Figure 9.8). The philtrum is usually short and the frontal teeth prominent. Assess the hands, as the fingers are usually tapering; retinal examination will often show pigmentary changes. In the newborn, prominence of the nasal bridge is exceptional. A high nasal bridge in an infant with unusual tone, poor feeding, or tremulousness suggestive of seizure activity could be the clue to **Wolf-Hirschhorn syndrome** (chromosome 4p deletion). Extreme flattening of the nasal bridge and midfacial region is seen in **chondrodysplasia punctata** and **in fetal warfarin embryopathy.** In the absence of warfarin exposure, clinical findings of limb asymmetry, ichthyosis, or patchy areas of rough skin with large pores, resembling orange peel, strongly suggest chondrodysplasia punctata. Patients with **Stickler syndrome,** an autosomal dominant condition, usually have depressed nasal bridge as a familial characteristic. Suspect Stickler syndrome as the underlying pathology in infants with Pierre-Robin sequence of cleft palate and micrognathia; in older children, excessive joint laxity, conductive deafness, myopia, and retinal detachment are regularly observed. It is worth observing the size of the joints, as large knees are a good clinical clue to the diagnosis of Stickler syndrome.

Investigations to Consider Unexplained granulocytopenia is often seen in Cohen syndrome and is a cheap diagnostic adjunct in clinically suspicious cases. Most 4p- cases are not seen on routine chromosome preparation and need specific FISH analysis for 4p16 band to confirm the diagnosis. Neonatal radiology is important in chondrodysplasia punctata as the epiphyseal stippling can be transient.

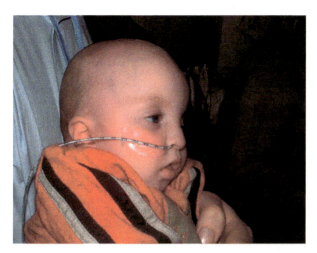

Figure 2.3A Note the prominent nasal bridge and glabellar region in this 9-month-old baby with Wolf-Hirschhorn syndrome. In this condition, the nose is sometimes described as having a "Greek helmet profile." The feeding tube betrays the continuing feeding difficulties.

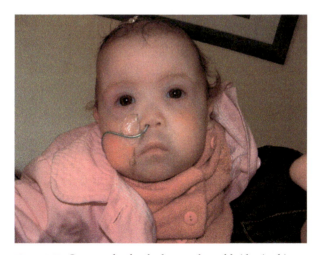

Figure 2.3B Contrast the deeply depressed nasal bridge in this picture with that in Figure 2.3A. The girl in this photograph shows epicanthic folds, especially noteworthy on the right, due to the nasal bridge depression. The underlying diagnosis in this case is chondrodysplasia punctata.

2.4 Abnormal Alae Nasi and Nasal Tip

Recognizing the Sign The alae nasi comprise the lateral walls of the nostrils, descending from the nasal tip to merge with the upper lip. In the event of hypoplasia, the nose acquires a pinched appearance. If combined with a wide nasal tip, the shape of the nose is described as cylindrical.

Establishing a Differential Diagnosis Prominence of the nasal tip with narrow ala nasi represents an excellent diagnostic clue and the examination must reflect this. Look at the hairline, which may be sparse temporally in **tricho-rhino-phalangeal (TRP) syndrome,** and seek a history of delayed hair growth in this scalp region. The hands usually show evidence of short metacarpals and the nails may be hypoplastic. As an autosomal dominant condition, assessment of other family members is important for supportive diagnostic signs. By contrast, a prominent nasal configuration against a background of hypocalcemia or congenital heart disease should prompt consideration of **velo-cardio-facial syndrome** (VCFS). Beware of the extreme variability of history and clinical findings in this disorder; a low threshold for investigation is advised. Nasal speech, delayed speech, a poor neonatal feeding history, and prolonged drooling may represent clues to pharyngeal incompetence, which attends many of these cases. The fingers are often long and hyperextensible. Absent joint skin crease of the fingers may be the clue to symphalangism, which, in the context of a large nasal tip and prominent nose should lead to examination of the wrists and ankles for carpal or tarsal fusion. An accompanying history of conductive deafness would seal a diagnosis of **WL symphalangism syndrome**, an autosomal dominant condition, justifying wider family inquiry and examination. Hypoplastic alae nasi with frontal upsweep of hair typify **Johanson-Blizzard syndrome** (Figure 1.6B), while notching of the alae nasi should prompt examination for lip pits, skin syndactyly, and knee webbing/pterygia, which are hallmarks of **Van der Woude syndrome**. Syndactyly, in the context of hypotelorism and hypoplastic alae nasi, signals oculodentodigital (ODD) syndrome (Figure 2.2).

Investigations to Consider FISH of 22q11 is the gold-standard investigation for VCFS, though if normal, 22q13 and 10p13 deletions may show clinical overlap. Extended cytogenetic band examination of chromosome 8q24 is warranted if TRP syndrome is clinically suspected, a deletion often being demonstrable. Mutation of the *NOG* gene underlies WL symphalangism but, like Van der Woude syndrome, the diagnosis is clinically identifiable in most cases.

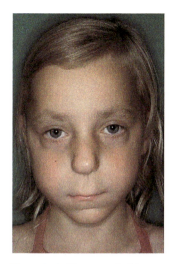

Figure 2.4A The nose of tricho-rhino-phalangeal syndrome is demonstrated. Note the bulbous tip and lack of alae nasi flare. There is relative prominence of the philtrum.

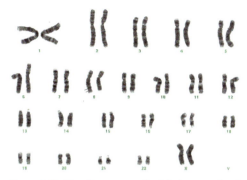

Figure 2.4B The chromosome 8q deletion associated with TRP syndrome is shown.

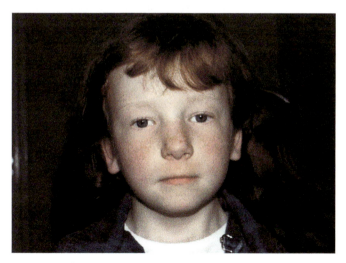

Figure 2.4C The nose in a patient with velo-cardio-facial syndrome, who presented with speech delay, aged 4 years. The tip is sometimes described as having a "square" appearance—as if it has been pinched, this aspect being seen especially well here.

2.5 Abnormal Nasal Columella and Nares

Recognizing the Sign The columella is the visible outer plane of the nasal septum, dividing the nostrils, whose aperture is the nares. The columella is usually situated at approximately the same level as the alae nasi and the nares not visualized. Should the length of the nose be reduced, then the columella slants from the foreshortened nasal tip and the nares become visible to frontal view, or "anteverted."

Establishing a Differential Diagnosis Anteverted nares do not necessarily signify an underlying syndromic diagnosis, but are particularly associated with a few well-established syndromes. **De Lange syndrome** will be recognizable by the characteristic synophrys of the eyebrows, low birth weight, short limbs, and, characteristically, short first metacarpal. Anteverted nares in **Williams syndrome** are often seen in the context of a neonatal cardiac murmur of supravalvular aortic stenosis, perhaps with documented hypercalcemia and a stellate pattern to the iris. Somewhat coarse features and hoarseness of the voice are typical of older Williams syndrome cases, but the anteversion of the nares remains a characteristic. Anteversion in a hyperteloric child and short stature are hallmark features of **Robinow syndrome**. Genital examination will often show micropenis in males, females being less noteworthy. In the newborn period gum hypertrophy can be a valuable sign to the diagnosis of Robinow syndrome. A different configuration, with extension of the columella below the alae nasi, is characteristic of **Rubinstein-Taybi syndrome**. Microcephaly and long eyelashes are associated facial characteristics but the clinical clue par excellence is broad thumbs and halluces, often deviated (Figure 9.12A). In **Floating-Harbor syndrome**, the columella is often similarly prominent, but the clinical background in this disorder is of short stature and mild developmental delay. Characteristically, the eyes are deep set. Prominence of the columella, with a full, rounded nasal tip, represents the quintessential description of the face in **Mowat-Wilson syndrome**, in which condition, severe developmental delay, often with microcephaly, and constipation define the clinical presentation. Other useful clinical signs include uplifted earlobes and an unusual vermillion border to the upper lip, which is full centrally but very thin at the outer aspects of the lip.

Investigations to Consider FISH of the *ELN* gene of chromosome 7q is indicated for Williams syndrome. Bone age delay is a sine qua non of Floating-Harbor, in which antigliadin antibodies and abnormal thyroid function should be sought. FISH is unrewarding in most cases of Rubinstein-Taybi syndrome, though mutation analysis is available in clinically doubtful instances. 2q22-23 deletions on karyotype typify a minority of Mowat-Wilson cases, with diagnosis relying on *ZFHX1B* mutation in all other instances.

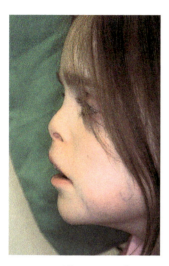

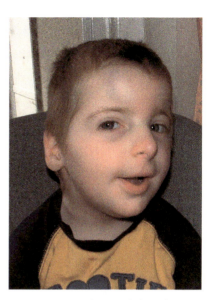

Figure 2.5A The anteverted nares of a patient with Robinow syndrome are demonstrated.

Figure 2.5B Note the rounded nasal tip and the columella extending below the level of the ala nasi in this patient who has Rubinstein-Taybi syndrome.

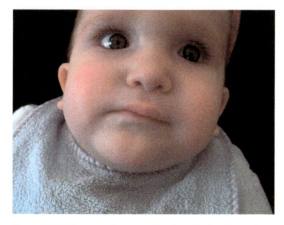

Figure 2.5C The prominent nasal columella in this patient in conjunction with the rounded nasal tip and the vermillion border of the upper lip demonstrating extreme thinning toward the margins of the mouth betray the diagnosis of Mowat-Wilson syndrome.

2.6 Abnormal Nasal Septum

Recognizing the Sign Shortening of the columella causes a flat nose but, provided the septum is straight, the nares are usually symmetric in shape. A half-moon configuration to the nares is commonly observed if the columella is short. A short columella is often associated with flattening of the nasal bridge, maxillary hypoplasia frequently accompanying and conferring a generally flat midfacial appearance. Deviation of the nasal septum results in asymmetric nares.

Establishing a Differential Diagnosis Flattening of the midface in a neonate should lead to inquiry as to intrapartum history, specifically relating to **environmental** and **teratogenic agents**. Fetal warfarin, fetal alcohol, and fetal rubella syndromes may all confer this presentation. A flat midface is also recorded in a few instances of infants born to mothers suffering systemic lupus erythematosus (SLE) during pregnancy, a further important aspect for specific historical inquiry. Nasal septum deviation and flattening of the nose is common in **oligohydramnios**, as a consequence of fetal constriction, of which other features such as arthrogryposis or cranial asymmetry should be sought. Older children with a flat nose and short septum are often termed as having **Binder syndrome**. The anterior nasal spine is missing and this can be palpated clinically by putting the finger inside the upper lip and pressing in the midline, at the base of the frenulum. Try it on yourself first, but the absence of this osseous landmark results in a soft, cartilaginous, mobile sensation. If absent, or in doubt, examine the patient's fingers. The nails are often small, reflecting an underlying hypoplasia of the terminal digits. Stature is often reduced, with symmetric limb shortening. As this can be familial, a family history can assist in demarcating from overlapping pathologies. A particular condition to be mindful of is **acrodysostosis**, an autosomal dominant form of short stature, in which relative macrocephaly and short fingers can lead to a clinical misdiagnosis of achondroplasia. The face in the older patient with acrodysostosis is sometimes described as "pugilistic." A short columella in a child with congenital heart disease or neonatal feeding difficulties may be indicative of **Kabuki syndrome** (Figure 3.14). Examination of the palpebral fissures for lower eyelid ectropion, of the lip for pits, and of the eyebrow for exaggerated arching or interruption would all lend diagnostic support.

Investigations to Consider Early x-rays often show epiphyseal stippling and suggest mutation of the X-linked *ARSE* gene in males with Binder syndrome. Cone-shaped epiphyses are characteristic of acrodysostosis.

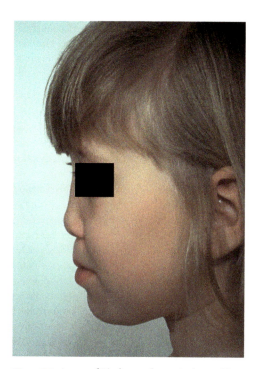

Figure 2.6 A case of Binder syndrome is shown. Note
the flat midface and shallow septum of the nose.
Viewed from beneath, the nares have a characteristic
half-moon shape.

2.7 Abnormal Nasal Appendages

Recognizing the Sign These signs are not the subject of clinical doubt. The nose itself is normally formed, the cause of clinical disquiet resting upon attendant features that are recognized as abnormal. Such may comprise a swelling at the base of the nose, a sinus, a polyp, a hair-bearing pit, or the emergence of papillomata around the nares.

Establishing a Differential Diagnosis Particularly if located in the midline, a sinus, whether hair bearing or blind ending, needs careful evaluation because of the possibility of direct communication to the central nervous system (CNS). In a neonate, observe the baby crying and specifically assess whether there is any swelling of the glabellar region, which may signify an **anterior encephalocele**. In addition, there are specific syndromic considerations. Careful evaluation of the upper lip and intraoral structures for **Pai syndrome** is indicated by the presence of a sinus or polyp. The upper lip may show minor midline clefting or upper frenulum reduplication. A pedunculated intraoral mass may be identified. Evidence of cleft palate or uvula should be sought. By contrast, the development of discrete lumpy masses around the nares, signifying nasal papillomata, typically being noted around 5 or 6 years of age, is strongly indicative of **Costello syndrome**. There will be a background history of severe failure to thrive following normal or slightly increased birth weight, merging into later concerns as to an underlying storage disease due to the developmental delay and coarse appearance of the patient. There is usually excess palmar skin with palmar and plantar hyperkeratosis, and the position of the fingers can show significant ulnar drift. Examine specifically for scoliosis. In the older patient, papules on the nose should provoke inquiry as to family history of breast or thyroid cancer. The concern is that the papules represent clues to a diagnosis of **Cowden syndrome**, an autosomal dominant cancer predisposition syndrome of broad clinical embrace. The examination should assess for macrocephaly and seek familial evidence for this feature. Examine for papules around the eyes, mouth, and upper lip, and intraorally. Likewise, palmoplantar keratosis supports this likely diagnosis, as does a rugosity of the tongue, sometimes described as "scrotal."

Investigations to Consider Nasal sinuses come with a low threshold for cranial neuroimaging to exclude associated encephalocele. Lipomata, sometimes of the corpus callosum, are frequent in Pai syndrome, but rarely impact adversely on CNS development. Rhabdomyosarcomata have been described in older Costello patients, and appropriate screening measures are recommended. The Cowden syndrome disease spectrum is best confirmed by *PTen* mutation analysis.

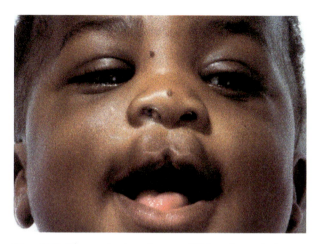

Figure 2.7A The nasal polyp of a case of Pai syndrome is demonstrated. Note the midline upper lip cleft and the sinus at the root of the nose.

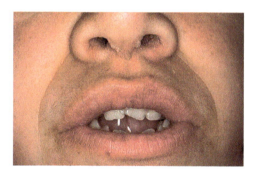

Figure 2.7B This photograph demonstrates the nasal papillomata of Costello syndrome, which only developed when the patient was 6 years old.

2.8 Synophrys

Recognizing the Sign Synophrys is the term used to describe eyebrows that meet in the midline over the nasal root. It is a normal finding in some individuals, but is seen more frequently in association with hypotelorism (see 2.2 and Figure 2.2A).

Establishing a Differential Diagnosis In the newborn period, noteworthy synophrys, particularly in a low-birth-weight infant, is an almost invariable finding in **de Lange syndrome.** The nasal bridge is usually depressed, the nares anteverted, the philtrum long, and the limbs short, with oligodactyly (absent fingers) in upward of a quarter of all cases. Even with no digital deficit, the hands have a characteristic appearance, the thumb being proximally inserted due to an underlying short first metacarpal (Figure 9.13B). In an older child with synophrys, a history of early normal milestones and then gradual developmental concern, often with unexplained diarrhea, should lead the examiner to consider **Sanfilippo syndrome**. Unlike other mucopolysaccharidoses, hepatosplenomegaly and other features of storage disorders including coarse facies, corneal clouding, and gingival thickening are often absent. An easily overlooked diagnosis, Sanfilippo syndrome is often flagged by parental accounts of behavioral concerns and worsening aggression but requires careful, targeted history taking. Synophrys, perhaps with associated flaring of the medial region of the eyebrows, is seen in some cases of **Waardenburg syndrome**, for which reason examination for pigmentary disturbance and telecanthus as well as clinical assessment of hearing are advised (Figure 2.1B). Frontal upsweep of the hair, male pseudohermaphroditism, and severe developmental delay in a patient with synophrys might cause **ATRX syndrome** to be considered as the underlying diagnosis. Likewise, a flat midface appearance or fleeting impression of a Down syndrome appearance are very common in the newly emerging **chromosome 9q34 microdeletion syndrome**. Besides synophrys, brachycephaly, macroglossia, and truncal hypotonia are other commonly observed clinical findings to be aware of in this diagnosis, as is the development of truncal obesity.

Investigations to Consider Classic de Lange syndrome is a clinical diagnosis. Cases of "mild" de Lange and atypical cases may need to have diagnosis confirmed molecularly by DNA analysis of the *NIPBL* gene on chromosome 5p. Bone age may be advanced in Sanfilippo syndrome, though features of dysostosis are not consistently present. Urinary mucopolysaccharides may be within normal range. Oligosaccharides may be increased, but enzymatic analysis in white cells or fibroblasts is usually reliable. 9q34 microdeletion syndrome requires comparative genome hybridization techniques in specialized laboratories for diagnosis. Waardenburg syndrome should be assessed audiologically. If molecular confirmation is required, *PAX3* analysis generally demonstrates mutation provided telecanthus is present.

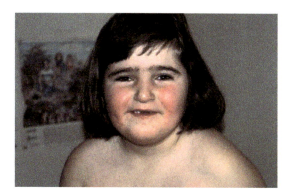

Figure 2.8 Synophrys is clearly seen in this patient, who has a diagnosis of Cohen syndrome, a condition not usually associated with synophrys. Note the prominent nasal bridge, narrow palpebral fissures, and short philtrum, which, in the context of her developmental delay, signal the diagnosis.

2.9 Midfacial Hypoplasia

Recognizing the Sign There is much scope for confusion here, the terms "malar hypoplasia," referring to the zygomatic region immediately below the eye, and "maxillary hypoplasia," referring to the immediately inferior region of the face, sometimes being used interchangeably. Essentially, this feature is present if the cheek bones are flat.

Establishing a Differential Diagnosis Check whether this is familial by observing facial characteristics of the parents. Midface hypoplasia is the hallmark of **Treacher Collins syndrome**, often with a tongue-shaped projection of scalp hair onto the cheek. Examine the ears, the pinnae of which are usually malformed, often with accompanying tags of skin or fistulae, and look for lower eyelid coloboma. As should always be undertaken in midface hypoplasia, an inspection of the palate will show clefting in about a third of Treacher Collins cases. Beware of the close resemblance in facial and even ear features to **Nager syndrome**, which is distinguished from Treacher Collins by the presence of radial hand malformations, including thumb hypoplasia. Concerns that early development is not proceeding normally, often associated with abnormalities of muscle tone or feeding problems in a baby whose appearance is not frankly dysmorphic but in whom midface hypoplasia is definitely present, may suggest the autosomal recessive disorder of **Schinzel-Giedion syndrome**. The forehead is tall and usually there is a noteworthy infraorbital skin groove (Figure 1.7B). Choanal stenosis occurs frequently and should be sought. An infraorbital skin crease is also an invaluable clinical sign in **fetal valproate syndrome**, running downward and laterally from the inner canthus region. Seek a confirmatory history of valproate exposure and, if confirmed, look further for metopic ridging and long philtrum. Preaxial polydactyly of the foot or thenar eminence hypoplasia are solid supportive signs, frequently not present but of strong diagnostic value if observed. Midface hypoplasia, with a smooth philtrum and thin upper lip, characterize **fetal alcohol syndrome**, though the history of fetal exposure can be harder to elicit. Look for aberrant skin creases of the hands, skin syndactyly of the fingers, short palpebral fissures, and poor growth, otherwise unexplained.

Investigations to Consider Deafness, usually conductive, is the norm in Treacher Collins cases. Mutation analysis is reserved for clinically subtle or doubtful cases, but demonstration of hypoplastic zygomatic processes on skull x-ray can obviate the need for DNA analysis. Computed tomography (CT) scan of the petrous temporal bone usually demonstrates ossicular malformations, consistent with a conductive deafness. Renal ultrasound demonstrating cysts or hydronephrosis would strongly support the likely diagnosis in Schinzel-Giedion syndrome. Demonstration of an occipital synchondrosis on skull x-ray is confirmatory.

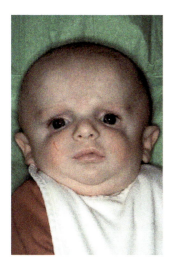

Figure 2.9A In this image of a patient with Treacher Collins syndrome, the zygomatic region immediately below the palpebral fissure is hypoplastic bilaterally.

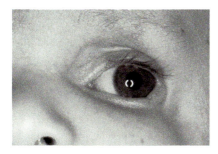

Figure 2.9B The characteristic lower eyelid coloboma of Treacher Collins syndrome is demonstrated in the same patient.

2.10 Micrognathia

Recognizing the Sign Best viewed in profile, this clinical sign is caused by a small mandible that has not grown out. When opening the lips, there is usually a malalignment of the alveolar margins in neonates and of the teeth in older patients. The chin is small or, in the adult patient, often grows out but may have a receding profile. Pierre-Robin sequence refers to a cleft palate consequent upon the posterior displacement of the tongue within the developing oral cavity occasioned by a primary failure of the mandible to advance.

Establishing a Differential Diagnosis In any case of Pierre-Robin sequence, **Stickler syndrome** should be a diagnostic concern, and evidence from the family history of high myopia, retinal detachment, early-onset arthropathy, or deafness would certainly strongly advance this diagnostic likelihood. Clinically, observe if the nasal bridge is depressed and look for excess joint laxity. Ophthalmic examination may show congenital cataract. Experienced ophthalmologists will specifically seek vitreous abnormalities. In other cases of micrognathia with cleft palate, examine the fingers. A misshapen index finger in a micrognathic patient, usually with ulnar deviation of that digit, is diagnostic of **Catel-Manzke syndrome**. Intelligence is generally normal in these cases, but there is a known association with cardiac defects, for which reason formal cardiac evaluation is indicated. Micrognathia as the striking facial feature of a child who has unexplained growth deficiency and a history of low birth weight may signify **Meier-Gorlin syndrome** (Figure 11.8). Confirmatory clinical support should be sought by palpating the patellae, which are absent, and by observing the ears, which are small. In contrast, children with **cerebro-costo-mandibular syndrome** will generally present with a Pierre-Robin picture at birth, often with associated respiratory problems, and emerging developmental concerns will cloud the clinical picture. Micrognathia is a nonspecific finding in many different forms of **chromosomal aneuploidy**. The author has personal experience of extreme micrognathia, requiring prolonged tracheotomy, as the sole presenting finding in patients who later proved to have chromosomal mosaicism. Accordingly, careful skin examination for areas of pigmentary differences and areas of localized keratosis pilaris and evaluation of skin under Wood's lamp is advised.

Investigations to Consider X-ray of the hands in Catel-Manzke syndrome will show an accessory metacarpal bone at the base of the index finger, while chest x-ray is the key to cerebrocostomandibular syndrome diagnosis, showing the discontinuity in rib outline, "rib gaps," diagnostic of the condition. Karyotype and even skin karyotype are indicated in cases without a recognized syndrome diagnosis in an attempt to formally exclude mosaicism.

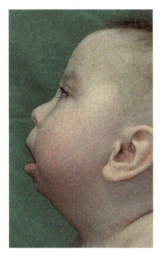

Figure 2.10A Micrognathia, requiring tracheostomy for airway maintenance, is shown in a patient with slightly coarse facial features and poor temporal hair growth at age 2 years. Wood's lamp examination showed streaky pigmentary disturbance consistent with chromosomal mosaicism. Karyotype from lymphocytes was normal, as was fibroblast karyotype. A second skin biopsy eventually demonstrated the chromosomal mosaicism. Keratinocyte culture is technically much more demanding and not routinely available for this reason, but is reported to have a higher yield in identifying occult mosaicism. See Figure 12.10 for Wood lamp skin findings in this same patient.

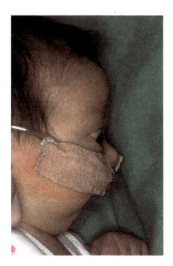

Figure 2.10B A typical micrognathic presentation is seen in this patient whose ophthalmic examination showed features consistent with Stickler syndrome.

2.11 Facial Asymmetry

Recognizing the Sign Some normal variation between the left and right sides of the face is to be anticipated. Neonatally, the clinician must be aware of the scope for facial asymmetry representing intrauterine forces, such as oligohydramnios, or normal molding in transit through the birth canal. Most such instances represent transient asymmetry and self-correct.

Establishing a Differential Diagnosis The possibility of an underlying **craniosynostosis** needs to be borne in mind (1.1), and a search for clinical signs of syndromic forms of craniosynostosis is worthwhile. As many are autosomal dominant, do observe the parental facial features. Broad thumbs and halluces are typical of Pfeiffer syndrome, while Apert syndrome is easily recognized through the extreme syndactyly ("mitten") of both hands and feet. Some mild skin syndactyly of fingers 3/4 is characteristic in Saethre-Chotzen syndrome. If **oligohydramnios** is suspected, look at the joints for limitation of movement and carefully observe the joint skin creases, their absence signifying paucity of movement in utero. Ear malformations in the context of facial asymmetry, such as microtia or preauricular skin tags, are likely to represent a diagnosis of **Goldenhar syndrome**. A parent may draw the clinician's attention to an infant whose face looks normal at rest but who, on crying, manifests significant facial asymmetry, especially around the mouth, which is typical of **asymmetric crying facies syndrome** (ACFS). The eye movement and eyelid closure are usually normal, the movement disorder being confined to the lower face. Careful examination of the heart for murmur and of the anus for stenosis is indicated in ACFS. Facial asymmetry with upper lip hemangioma is characteristic of the **macrocephaly-cutis marmorata-telangiectasia congenita (MCTC) syndrome**, in which condition, 2/3 toe syndactyly, limb asymmetry, and delayed development should be anticipated (Figure 12.12). In the absence of hemangiomata, lipomata, or other cutaneous manifestations, facial asymmetry with accompanying limb asymmetry is usually classed as **isolated hemihyperplasia**. Such children generally have normal developmental outcomes, but screening for Wilms tumor is advocated, certainly until the age of 7 years. Evolving facial asymmetry in an older child is characteristic of **Parry-Romberg syndrome**, in which a history of a previously symmetric face is usual. There is a progressive hemifacial atrophy, often affecting the scalp with localized areas of hair loss.

Investigations to Consider Skull radiology should be undertaken to look for sutural synostosis if craniosynostosis is suspected. Vertebral x-rays are important in Goldenhar syndrome to assess for hemivertebrae. ACFS overlaps clinically with deletion 22q.11 syndrome and FISH for this deletion is appropriate, as is differential white cell count. Transient hypocalcemia has been observed occasionally.

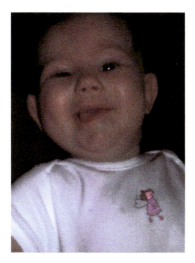

Figure 2.11A This baby has asymmetric crying facies syndrome. There is very little movement on the left side of the face on opening the mouth, smiling or crying.

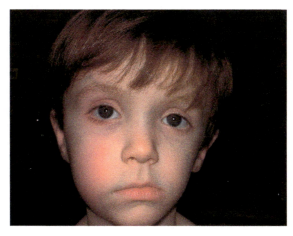

Figure 2.11B Right-sided facial hemihyperplasia in an otherwise normal 5-year-old is shown.

2.12 Myopathic Facies

Recognizing the Sign Poor muscle tone of the facial muscles results in a somewhat narrow face. Often the clue to a muscle pathology is fairly obvious, there being drooling, poor feeding, or swallowing and ptosis.

Establishing a Differential Diagnosis Ptosis in infancy can be difficult to elicit; remember to sit the baby upright before concluding that this sign is absent. Many children with weak facial musculature have an underlying **primary muscle disease**, in consequence of which general muscle bulk, tone, reflexes, and observations on handling the baby are all of potential significance. Likewise, family history may be invaluable and hold the key to the diagnosis. **Myotonic dystrophy** represents a case in point, the congenitally affected infant frequently having a history of polyhydramnios but the signs in the mother being more subtle and requiring formal questioning and/or examination to elicit the characteristic myotonia. The best objective clinical test in such females is percussion of the thenar eminence, with the thumb failing to relax back across the hand but staying in the cross-palmar position for a few minutes due to the myotonia. **Mitochondrial disease** may also cause facial muscle weakness, and a family history consistent with mitochondrial inheritance may be pertinent. A maternal history of squint or epilepsy should not be discounted. The signature of **Moebius syndrome** is facial weakness characterized by congenital bilateral sixth and seventh nerve palsy. However, since bulbar involvement is common, examination of the lower cranial nerves is no less important. Continue the examination by careful attention to the upper limbs; brachydactyly, syndactyly, and oligodactyly are consistent with the Moebius diagnosis. The chest wall musculature should be formally examined, particularly the pectoralis major, the sternal head of which may be deficient in Moebius syndrome. Cleft palate is also described in Moebius syndrome, but cleft palate and myopathic facies are more likely to signify a distinct autosomal recessive condition, **Carey-Fineman-Ziter syndrome**. In the event of this syndrome being considered, a good clinical sign to look for is the presence of dimples at the wrist. Myopathic facies in a tall male with arachnodactyly and a marfanoid habitus but who is developmentally delayed is typical of the rare X-linked condition, **Lujan-Fryns syndrome**.

Investigations to Consider If a primary muscle disease is suspected, muscle biopsy, specialized staining, and targeted DNA investigation will likely form the basis of diagnosis. For myotonic dystrophy, expansion of the triplet repeat mutation is confirmatory of the clinical findings. Specialized staining with Gomori trichrome of muscle, muscle enzyme biochemistry, and mitochondrial DNA analysis may be required to confirm mitochondrial disease.

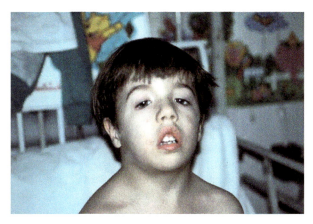

Figure 2.12 A typical example of a patient with myopathic facies. Note the downslanting palpebral fissures, bilateral ptosis, facial weakness, and sloping shoulders. (Reproduced with permission of Wiley-Liss from Baraitser and Reardon, *Am J Med Genet* 1994; 53:163–164.)

2.13 Abnormalities of the Philtrum

Recognizing the Sign The philtrum occupies that region of the upper lip between the nasal columella and the vermilion of the lip. The appearance of the philtrum is governed to some extent by the relationship to the nose, a short nose resulting in a long philtrum and vice versa. Considered in isolation, characteristics of the philtrum rarely represent signatures of specific syndromes, but observations of the philtrum can consolidate and support additional clinical findings to cumulatively suggest a likely clinical diagnosis.

Establishing a Differential Diagnosis Though perhaps the most celebrated, **fetal alcohol syndrome** (FAS) is not the only cause of a smooth philtrum, the philtral pillars being indistinct. However, this appearance is seen in many children with a firm history of excess alcohol exposure in utero. Even if the antenatal history is not immediately forthcoming, a low birth weight; poor postnatal growth; short palpebral fissures, perhaps with a degree of ptosis; and a thin upper lip may suggest the diagnosis. Optic nerve hypoplasia should be sought, and retinal arterial tortuosity, if observed, will further consolidate the diagnosis. Clinical evidence of radioulnar or carpal synostosis is worth seeking, as is partial syndactyly of the fingers and abnormal palmar crease patterns (Figure 9.18D). Remember that a short and smooth philtrum in the context of unexplained growth failure is also characteristic of **Floating-Harbor syndrome**. Celiac disease or hypothyroidism would consolidate the latter condition as the more likely diagnosis. Both **Robinow syndrome** and **Aarskog syndrome** are further short stature syndromes associated with noteworthy philtral features, being long in Robinow syndrome and wide in Aarskog syndrome (Figure 2.1A). The key to the correct diagnosis is genital examination, the scrotum being shawl shaped in Aarskog syndrome and there being micropenis in Robinow syndrome. In **fetal valproate syndrome** the philtrum is generally long and smooth, the most characteristic facial finding being the infraorbital skin crease. The rather bulbous nose of tricho-rhino-phalangeal (**TRP**) **syndrome**, particularly accentuated by the ala nasi hypoplasia, draws the examiner's eye, giving the impression of a prominent philtrum. The philtrum of **Cohen syndrome** is typically short (Figure 2.8). Prominent incisors, a high nasal bridge, narrow palpebral fissures, developmental delay, and truncal obesity combine to suggest this autosomal recessive diagnosis. Examination of the hands generally shows long, tapering fingers, perhaps with some excess joint laxity.

Investigations to Consider Delayed bone age is common to both FAS and Floating-Harbor syndromes, the diagnosis being clinical in both instances. Chromosomal examination, specifically of 8q24, may disclose a localized deletion in TRP syndrome. Granulocytopenia is a useful supportive clue to the diagnosis of Cohen syndrome.

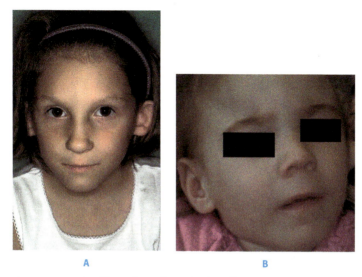

A   B

Figure 2.13A and B The patients shown in these illustrations both demonstrate smooth philtrum and thin upper lip, in both these instances associated with fetal alcohol syndrome. Prominence of the philtrum is well demonstrated in Figure 2.4A, a wide philtrum is shown in Figure 2.1A, and a short philtrum is exemplified by Figure 2.8.

Chapter 3　The Eye and Related Structures

3.1 Epicanthus

Recognizing the Sign Epicanthus refers to a vertical fold of redundant skin between the eye and the nose, originating below the eye and extending upward, eventually blending with the upper lid, the inner canthus occasionally being obscured by this skin fold.

Establishing a Differential Diagnosis Epicanthus is a normal finding in many infants, due to a depressed nasal bridge, and will usually disappear by the second birthday, as the nasal bridge develops. Family history can be important, with surgery for ptosis in a parent suggesting **blepharophimosis-ptosis-epicanthus inversus syndrome** (BPES). Infertility in adult females in the family is another useful clue to this disorder. The associated presence of ptosis, often with compensatory frontalis muscle overactivity giving transverse creasing of the forehead, is a useful clinical sign to observe. Likewise, look for a compensatory backward tilt of the head. The palpebral fissure may be somewhat short and, in a minority of cases, there can be developmental delay. Be aware that some children can be diagnosed with developmental delay prematurely and surgical intervention for ptosis can result in developmental catch-up. Epicanthic folds are well known through the association with **Down syndrome**, but are nonspecifically observed in a whole range of chromosomal aneuploidies, all of which will give rise to developmental concerns. Epicanthus persisting into late childhood and beyond is characteristic of **Stickler syndrome**, due to the depressed nasal bridge, so do check for cleft palate repair, excess joint laxity, and a history of retinal detachment. Other connective tissue associations to bear in mind when observing epicanthus include **Ehlers-Danlos syndrome** (EDS), in particular types I, II, and VI. Excess joint laxity, scarring in response to minor skin trauma, keloid formation, skin hyperextensibility, prominent nasolabial folds, and a generally "jowly" appearance are important clinical clues, as is the family history. Patients with **Williams syndrome** frequently have epicanthus. The neonatal presentation with murmur and hypercalcemia is easily diagnosed, but the later presentation with only slight developmental concerns can be deceiving. The best clinical clues in the older age group are hoarseness of voice with periorbital fullness and a stellate pattern to the iris (Figure 3.13).

Investigations to Consider In the presence of abnormal tone, concerns that there may be delayed development, or feeding difficulties, epicanthus most likely is a harbinger of a chromosomal aneuploidy and karyotyping is mandatory. For Williams syndrome, demonstration of a 7q deletion by fluorescence in situ hybridization (FISH) of *ELN* is diagnostic. A small number of cases of BPES have chromosome 3q23 deletions, but most are due to mutation within the *FOXL2* gene in this cytogenetic region.

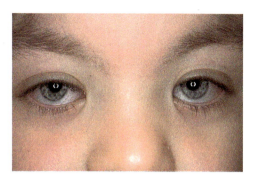

Figure 3.1 Epicanthus with associated mild bilateral ptosis is demonstrated in this 3-year-old child. Note also the nonspecific finding of lateral flaring of the eyebrows.

3.2 Deep-Set Eyes

Recognizing the Sign An important sign, deep-set eyes are frequently the harbinger of wider concerns. The neonate generally opens his or her eyes voluntarily in the first day or two of life. Failure to do so may reflect photophobia or underlying eye malformation, such as microphthalmia. Tightly shut eyes, which require a speculum to expose the eye, are typical of deep-set eyes and should prompt a formal pediatric ophthalmologic evaluation. Deep-set eyes are best appreciated by viewing the face from the side. The usual bulge created by the globe is reduced in volume and there is often an associated skin crease extending laterally from the margin of the palpebral fissure.

Establishing a Differential Diagnosis In a neonate, convincingly deep-set eyes must prompt specific examination. Think of **Freeman-Sheldon syndrome**, in which microstomia and camptodactyly of the hands are the clinical giveaway features (Figure 5.1), and **Rubinstein-Taybi syndrome**, in which the broad thumbs and prominent nasal columella should secure the clinical diagnosis. Secure that you have clinically excluded these two recognizable phenotypes, consider now two specific genetic conditions, Lowe syndrome and chromosome 1p36 deletion. **Lowe syndrome** is an X-linked condition of mental retardation, renal tubulopathy, and cataract, often associated with glaucoma. Hence, family history is important, as are urinary investigation for nonspecific aminoaciduria and ophthalmologic evaluation. Female carriers generally have cortical opacities of no visual significance identifiable on slit lamp examination. In contrast, **chromosome 1p36 deletion** is the second most common microdeletion syndrome after 22q11. Look for low-set or horizontal eyebrows with loss of normal arched shape. Unexplained obesity is a frequent observation. The helices of the ears should be examined for asymmetry, thickening of the helices, or pinna malformations. Hypotonia, neonatal feeding concerns, or delayed motor milestones in a child with deep-set eyes should stimulate specific investigation for this condition. **Lenz microphthalmia syndrome** classically presents with deep-set eyes. Inherited in X-linked dominant manner, a family history of coloboma, lens surgery, or retinal detachment offers valuable diagnostic support. Oligodontia should be sought in adult cases, and occasional skeletal features such as radioulnar synostosis or polydactyly are within the spectrum of malformations expected.

Investigations to Consider In Lowe syndrome be aware of the initial absence of aminoaciduria in urine during the neonatal period and repeat urinalysis after a few months. Elevated urinary retinol binding protein is the best single screening measure. Chromosome 1p36 deletions need specific cytogenetic analysis by targeted subtelomere studies, so discuss your clinical concerns with your laboratory. Lenz microphthalmia can be confirmed by mutation analysis of the *BCOR* gene on Xp27.

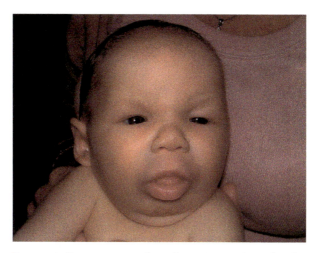

Figure 3.2A Deep-set eyes are shown in a patient aged 6 weeks, who did not open his eyes spontaneously for the first 2 weeks of life. Note also the slight telecanthus and mild degree of macroglossia.

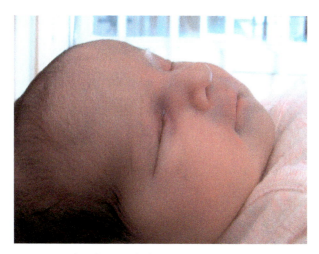

Figure 3.2B This photograph shows a 2-week-old baby girl with Lenz microphthalmia, whose deep-set eyes are readily appreciated in the lateral view. Note the skin crease lateral to the palpebral fissure.

3.3 Almond-Shaped Eyes

Recognizing the Sign The almond comparison is a good one. Palpebral fissure dimensions, the length of the palpebral fissure from the inner canthus to the outer canthus of each eye, may be reduced, giving a false clinical impression of microphthalmia, with the size of the globe being normal.

Establishing a Differential Diagnosis The almond-shaped eye sign is quintessentially associated with **Prader-Willi syndrome,** and the description of a palpebral fissure as being almond shaped must lead to evaluation of the other clinical aspects of this condition. In the neonate, hypotonia, poor sucking, transient need of special feeding techniques, and a history of reduced fetal movement are frequently recorded in Prader-Willi syndrome patients. The skull shape is often dolichocephalic, the upper lip may be thin, and the mouth may be small, with downturned corners. None of these signs is definitive but, in combination and with a supportive history, may well be signaling a diagnosis of Prader-Willi syndrome. Examine the genitalia; undescended testes and reduced penile length are well described in the male. Emerging developmental concerns and failure to achieve motor milestones are to be expected. Weight gain is a later feature but is always present by 6 years, usually associated with hyperphagia and food-related obsessional behavior. Other clinical clues that can be very useful are small hands and feet and a straight ulnar border to the hands; it is worth asking the parents whether the child picks at his or her skin, particularly at minor skin lesions. On direct questioning, a history of excess daytime sleeping may be forthcoming. The other main condition to consider in relation to this clinical sign is **chromosome 1p36 deletion**, in which asymmetric, sometimes thickened ear helices are good clinical clues, as are the eyebrows, which are somewhat horizontal with little by way of normal arching. Severe hypotonia neonatally and developmental delay in the older child are characteristic, with many affected individuals also having congenital heart disease of no specific diagnostic association.

Investigations to Consider Careful cytogenetic analysis is the approach to chromosome 1p36 deletion; specific subtelomere FISH or array hybridization are required if no deletion is microscopically visible in cases of strong clinical suspicion. Prader-Willi syndrome shows 15q11-13 deletion of the paternal chromosome in about 70% of cases. Uniparental maternal disomy of 15q11-13 accounts for 25% and requires DNA analysis of the patient and parents for confirmation.

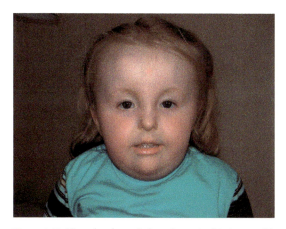

Figure 3.3A Note the almond-shaped eyes in this 2-year-old girl with confirmed Prader-Willi syndrome. The initial presentation in this girl was of neonatal feeding problems, requiring nasogastric intubation for several weeks. Neurologic evaluation confirmed hypotonia and muscle biopsy was suggestive of a congenital myopathy. After the age of 1 year, the rapid weight gain and global developmental concerns gave the clues to the true diagnosis.

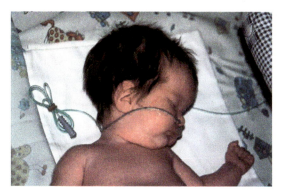

Figure 3.3B A typical neonatal presentation of Prader-Willi syndrome is pictured. Note the nasogastric feeding requirement and the dolichocephaly.

3.4 Blepharophimosis

Recognizing the Sign The clinical impression is of small eyes, but the globe is structurally and functionally normal in most instances. Blepharophimosis or short palpebral fissure, as it is also called, is a reduction of palpebral fissure length in the horizontal axis, measured from the inner canthus to the outer canthus of one eye. If present, this is generally bilateral. Ophthalmologic evaluation may reveal associated microphthalmia.

Establishing a Differential Diagnosis Observe the parents and obtain a family history of any surgery for ptosis. The autosomal dominant condition of **blepharophimosos-ptosis-epicanthus inversus syndrome** (BPES) tends to restrict the palpebral fissure, and such a finding in another family member is probably of diagnostic significance. Examine for epicanthus and ptosis. Observe the head position carefully for signs of the latter. In the absence of a family or suggestive history of BPES, examine the rest of the face. Look for micrognathia and cleft palate. These features may indicate a likely diagnosis of **Catel-Manzke syndrome**, in which blepharophimosis is typical. The clinching of this diagnosis will be by observation of the hands and seeing the unusual shape of the index fingers, which generally show ulnar deviation bilaterally. This is caused by an accessory metacarpal bone in the index fingers. Blepharophimosis may be a nonspecific indicator of chromosomal aneuploidies, particularly if associated with malformations, such as congenital heart disease, for which reason clinical evaluation of the heart is important. There are a few rare but diagnosable conditions in which blepharophimosis is characteristic and consequently merit specific consideration—**Hallermann-Streiff syndrome** presents a thin, prominent, and pointed nose; small chin; and small palpebral fissures. Neonatal cataracts or microphthalmia are almost universal. Short palpebral fissures are seen in many cases of **fetal alcohol syndrome**, in which the outer and inner canthi may be displaced toward the midline. Ptosis and/or epicanthus may be present also, but look for other clues such as a smooth philtrum, a thin upper lip, and aberrant creases of the palms and forearms. A history of low birth weight is usual.

Investigations to Consider A routine karyotype, without need for specific cytogenetic refinements, is appropriate if a generic "chromosomal" basis is to be excluded. Specifically, chromosome 3q23 abnormality should be sought in BPES, particularly if there is developmental delay, which may signify an associated loss of other genetic material by deletion of adjacent loci. Most BPES cases show intragenic mutation of the *FOXL2* gene on 3q23 by DNA analysis. Hand radiology demonstrating the accessory metacarpal bones of the index fingers is confirmatory of Catel-Manzke syndrome.

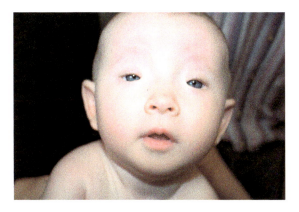

Figure 3.4A The classic signs of BPES comprising blepharophimosis, ptosis, and epicanthus inversus are readily appreciated.

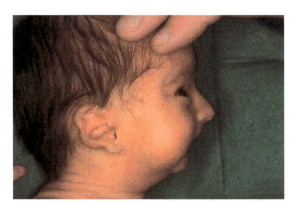

Figure 3.4B In profile, the micrognathia, beaked nose of blepharophimosis of this baby with Hallermann-Streigg syndrome are appreciated.

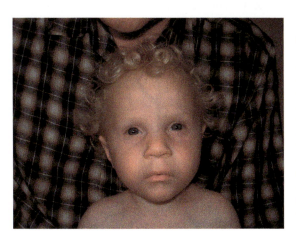

Figure 3.4C Short palpebral fissures are demonstrated in this boy with fetal alcohol syndrome. Note the clinical impression of small eyes. There is microcephaly and malar hypoplasia. Unlike many other cases of this disorder, the philtral pillars are quite well formed and the upper lip is not thin. Other diagnostically useful signs in this patient were partial 3/4 finger syndactyly and abnormal palmar creases.

3.5 Palpebral Fissure Slant

Recognizing the Sign Should the outer canthi be sited above an imaginary line connecting the two inner canthi, then the palpebral fissures slant upward (mongoloid); below such an imaginary line, the palpebral fissures slant downward (antimongoloid). Some variation is observed in up to 5% of the normal population.

Establishing a Differential Diagnosis Upslanting palpebral fissures suggest reduced skull growth relative to the midface, so assessment for microcephaly and associated signs is sensible (1.2). Apart from the well-established association with **Down syndrome**, upslanting palpebral fissures are a nonspecific finding in many cases of chromosomal aneuploidy. Of more specific diagnostic value, this sign is frequently seen in **Pallister-Killian syndrome**, tetrasomy chromosome 12p, in which condition additional clinical signs to look for are temporal balding, with poor hair growth in this region, and severe developmental delay. Accessory nipples and regional skin pigmentation abnormalities are important diagnostically supportive clinical signs, but not universally present. With age, affected patients develop a coarse appearance, reminiscent of storage disorders. Upslanting palpebral fissures are often noted in early childhood in **Kabuki syndrome**, the other ophthalmic signs being ectropion of the lower eyelid and hairless "gaps" in the eyebrows. Downslanting palpebral fissures frequently accompany midface hypoplasia and are common in conditions thus characterized. If the striking characteristic of a face is downslanting palpebral fissures, think specifically of **Noonan syndrome** and examine the heart; assess for familial short stature and low hairline on the neck, and ask about a personal or family history of bleeding disorders, as many Noonan cases have an unexplained coagulopathy. Downslanting palpebral fissures with associated hypertelorism and developmental delay in a male suggest **Coffin-Lowry syndrome** (Figure 9.9), especially if a history compatible with X-linked mental retardation can be established. Carrier females may show mild clinical signs. Particularly useful clinical signs to seek are rather full lips and tapering, fleshy fingers. The face of **Robinow syndrome** may also show hypertelorism and downslanting palpebral fissures, but there is usually little cause for developmental concern. Look specifically for gum hypertrophy and tongue tie, both valuable clues to this diagnosis, and, in males, for micropenis. The nose is usually anteverted and there is short stature.

Investigations to Consider Pallister-Killian syndrome patients almost invariably need fibroblast analysis to establish the diagnosis and, in some instances, need repeated skin biopsies to achieve this. Keratinocyte culture, rarely available, has a better yield. Spinal radiology is important in Robinow syndrome to assess for hemivertebrae or fusions, which may necessitate surgical management.

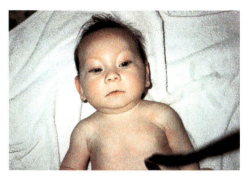

Figure 3.5A The upslant of the palpebral fissures in this baby with Kabuki syndrome is beyond dispute.

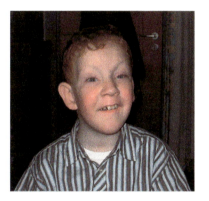

Figure 3.5B This photograph shows mildly upslanting palpebral fissures in a 13-year-old boy with Pallister-Killian syndrome.

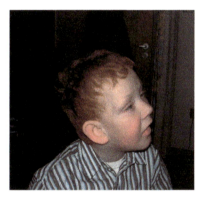

Figure 3.5C **The same patient is demonstrated as in Figure 3.5B.** Seen in profile, the temporal balding, typical of Pallister-Killian syndrome, has been minimized by brushing the hair forward onto the hairless region.

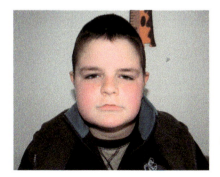

Figure 3.5D A striking example of downslanting palpebral fissures is shown.

3.6 Proptosis

Recognizing the Sign The globe of the eye protrudes inordinately. It is possible to measure the degree of orbital protrusion, but this is rarely undertaken in practice. A clinical impression of inordinate prominence of the eyes will lead the clinician to consider this sign and its related conditions.

Establishing a Differential Diagnosis First establish whether the proptosis is unilateral or bilateral. In craniosynostosis the premature fusion of the skull base causes reduced orbital volume and proptosis. With the exception of unicoronal synostosis, the proptosis is bilateral, even if asymmetric. Proptosis is the abiding clinical memory of the clinician's first glance at **Crouzon syndrome**. The absence of significant digital features on hand and foot examination will establish Crouzon syndrome as the likely diagnosis, while broad halluces and thumbs in the context of proptosis and clinical evidence of craniosynostosis on skull palpation will point toward **Pfeiffer syndrome**. **Apert syndrome** patients, readily recognizable by the syndactyly of fingers and toes, tend to have less significant degrees of proptosis than Crouzon syndrome, but do remember to look for cleft palate seen in 75% of Apert cases. By contrast, unilateral proptosis should prompt the astute clinician to examine the child for clinical signs of **neurofibromatosis type 1** (NF1). Specifically look for café-au-lait patches and macrocephaly. Observe if the eye is pulsatile, usually reflecting a deficiency of the greater wing of the sphenoid bone in the orbital wall. Peripheral neuromas, plexiform neuromas, and axillary and groin freckling should all be sought in the older child. It is important to examine for scoliosis and for hypertension, in view of the known association with renal artery stenosis and with pheochromocytoma. Bilateral eye prominence is also seen in some forms of **Ehlers-Danlos Syndrome** (EDS). Further clues to this condition may emerge from the family history. Examine the skin and joints for hyperlaxity. Look for evidence of bruising or exaggerated response to minimal trauma. An important clinical feature to establish is scoliosis, which generally signifies type VI, in which there is a propensity to perforation of the globe and retinal detachment.

Investigations to Consider Mutation analysis of the appropriate FGFR (Fibroblast Growth Factor Receptor) locus will usually offer molecular confirmation of a specific clinical syndrome of craniosynostosis. Slit lamp examination for Lisch nodules on the iris and retinal examination for signs of optic glioma are important elements of the assessment of NF1 in childhood. In EDS type VI, lysyl hydroxylase deficiency may be demonstrated on fibroblasts, but an easier screening test is to undertake urinary pyridinoline cross-links.

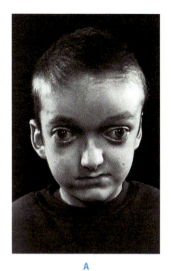 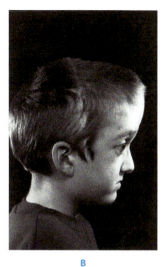

A   B

Figure 3.6A and B Proptosis is demonstrated in frontal (**A**) and lateral (**B**) views of a scaphocephalic patient who has a mutation of the *FGFR2* gene.

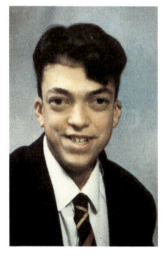

Figure 3.6C This photograph shows a classical case of Crouzon syndrome, demonstrating prop-tosis and hypertelorism.

3.7 Ptosis of the Eyelid

Recognizing the Sign The upper eyelid normally covers 2 cm of cornea, which approximates with the outer margin of the iris. Hence, sclera is usually not seen between the iris and the upper lid and, if present, suggests lid retraction. The eyes are wide open, sometimes described as "startled" appearance. Conversely, ptosis of the eyelid narrows the palpebral fissure.

Establishing a Differential Diagnosis Establish whether the ptosis is unilateral or bilateral and whether it is congenital or of later onset. Observe any compensatory head tilt of frontalis muscle overactivity. **Blepharophimosis-ptosis-epicanthus inversus syndrome** (BPES) has already been outlined (2.1). Affected individuals do not manifest all the signs in all cases, so family history allied with careful examination will be useful in diagnosis of this autosomal dominant condition. Establish whether the patient has the full range of eye movements and examine the cranial nerves. Evidence of VI and VII nerve palsy, often with signs of more extensive lower cranial nerve deficiencies, suggests a likely diagnosis of **Moebius syndrome** and attention should be given to the hands—syndactyly or brachydactyly being common in this condition. Clinical awareness, neurologic history and physical signs are the key to diagnosis of the **mitochondrial myopathies**, in which conditions the gradual development of ptosis with age is common. A family history, particularly with attention to symptoms in the maternal lineage, may offer clues, though many cases are sporadic. Examine for ophthalmoplegia and general muscle weakness. Seek a history of stroke-like episodes or myoclonic epilepsy. Ptosis in association with short stature and/or a cardiac murmur may be the signals to a case of **Noonan syndrome**. Look for a low posterior hairline and evidence of excess nuchal skin, which will further support this diagnosis, if present. Often seen in **Saethre-Chotzen type craniosynostosis**, the true nature of the ptosis is betrayed by the unusually upright forehead shape, prominent ear crus, and partial skin syndactyly of the fingers. The frequent observation of ptosis in the condition of **Wilms-aniridia-genital abnormality-retardation** (WAGR) emphasizes the need for careful ophthalmic and general evaluation of the patient with ptosis in the interest of the true diagnosis emerging. Cryptorchidism and hypospadias are useful clinical prompts in cases of WAGR syndrome.

Investigations to Consider Investigation of mitochondrial myopathies includes electrocardiogram (ECG) for block, audiologic evaluation for deafness, and retinal examination for pigmentary retinopathy. Muscle biopsy for ragged red fibers by Gomori trichrome stain may be indicated. Mitochondrial DNA study for deletions/duplications or point mutations may be valuable. Karyotype usually shows 11p13 deletion in WAGR, whereas karyotype in BPES may show 3q deletion.

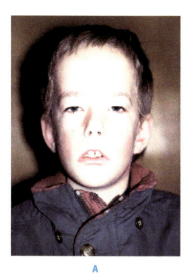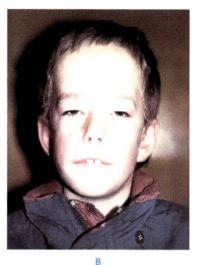

A	B

Figure 3.7A and B Bilateral ptosis is demonstrated in a patient with Moebius syndrome of bilateral facial diplegia. The paucity of facial movement is demonstrated between the facial expression at rest (**A**) and smiling (**B**). Note the degree to which the upper eyelid obscures the iris and pupil. Additionally, the upper eyelid crease is absent, a further sign of ptosis. (Reproduced with permission of Wiley-Liss from Reardon et al., *Am J Med Genet* 2003;122A:84–88.)

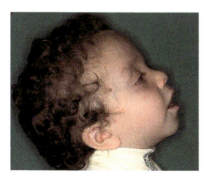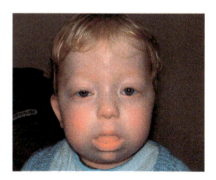

Figure 3.7C This photograph shows ptosis in a patient with Noonan syndrome; observe the compensatory backward tilt of the head.

Figure 3.7D This photograph demonstrates unilateral ptosis. Note also the macroglossia in this boy.

3.8 Corneal Clouding

Recognizing the Sign A generalized hazy appearance of the cornea is present, usually bilaterally. Specific forms of corneal clouding are described, most notably buphthalmos ("bull's eye"), in which congenital glaucoma causes enlargement of the anterior chamber and cloudy cornea. Sclerocornea is a term used in describing congenital, nonprogressive corneal opacification.

Establishing a Differential Diagnosis Formal ophthalmologic evaluation is essential in determining the likely cause and management of corneal clouding. Essentially, three main causes should be considered: (1) glaucoma; (2) primary anterior eye chamber diseases, which sometimes have other clinical manifestations; and (3) metabolic disease. While **glaucoma** is well described in Sturge-Weber and Rubinstein-Taybi syndromes, the corneal clouding is not the primary clinical finding in such instances and the underlying diagnosis is evident from the characteristic facial hemangioma of the former and broad, deviated thumbs and characteristic nasal columella of the latter. Likewise, congenital glaucoma can be seen in Stickler syndrome, other clues to the true diagnosis coming from the enlarged joints, excess joint laxity, and cleft palate, if present, in addition to the family history. Most glaucoma is nonsyndromic and nonocular signs will not be established. Among **primary anterior eye chamber disorders**, clinical clues to such a diagnosis will be eccentric siting of the pupil or absence of the iris. Extended neonatal jaundice in an infant with cloudy cornea should highlight the diagnostic likelihood of **Alagille syndrome**. The finding of congenital heart disease, particularly peripheral pulmonary stenosis, would support this diagnosis. **Rieger syndrome** presents with congenital iris dysplasia, often resulting in glaucoma. The clinical clues to the diagnosis lie in the frequent history of anal stenosis, hypodontia, the incisors often being absent, and failure of involution of umbilical skin, frequently resulting in surgery for umbilical hernia. Ptosis, cryptorchidism, and hypospadias will signal **WAGR** (Wilm's Tumor, Aniridia, Genitalia Retardation) syndrome, while a family history of autosomal dominant anterior chamber anomalies is often available on inquiry in isolated aniridia cases. Corneal clouding in **biochemical diseases** can represent mucopolysaccharidosis, mucolipidosis, or gangliosidosis. Useful clinical clues may comprise organomegaly, gum hypertrophy, developmental delay, and short stature.

Investigations to Consider If Alagille syndrome is suspected, look for hemivertebrae or butterfly vertebrae radiologically and get an echocardiograph. In WAGR, chromosome 11p deletions should be sought, but basic karyotype is warranted in the absence of a specific ophthalmic diagnosis. *PAX6* gene mutation analysis may be valuable in isolated/familial cases of anterior chamber malformations without signs of Rieger syndrome. Increased urinary mucopolysaccharides, oligosaccharides, and vacuolated lymphocytes on blood smear are appropriate basic screening measures for biochemical conditions.

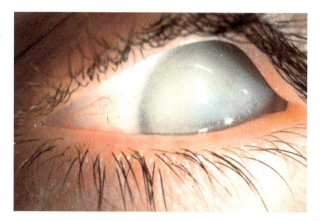

Figure 3.8 This photograph shows corneal clouding in a patient with mucopolysaccharidosis. (Courtesy of Dr. Paul Connell.)

3.9 Ectopic Pupil

Recognizing the Sign Usually central within the iris, eccentric siting of the pupil is visible on inspection of the eye, generally affecting both eyes, though there may be asymmetry in the degree of involvement. In extreme cases, the displacement of the pupil may give the clinical appearance of iris coloboma.

Establishing a Differential Diagnosis As applies to corneal clouding, formal ophthalmologic evaluation is mandatory to establish the primary diagnosis for this clinical sign. Be aware that there may be associated underlying lens dislocation, cataracts, or retinal detachment. In many cases the clinical signs are confined to the eye. It is worth taking a family history, as there are sibships reported with ectopic pupils, often associated with lens and other anterior chamber malformations. In conducting the rest of the clinical examination, particular reference to those conditions, already outlined in relation to corneal clouding, that cause anterior chamber malformations is advised. Specifically, look for a history of extended neonatal jaundice or established bile duct paucity on histologic examination in **Alagille syndrome** or in such a patient who also has a cardiac murmur. Seek the history of anal stenosis, often requiring surgical intervention, or surgical treatment for umbilical "hernia," which may betray the diagnosis of **Rieger syndrome**. Since these are autosomal dominant disorders, an extended family history may uncover other, previously unremarked upon, valuable corroborative evidence of either diagnosis. In **Peter's anomaly**, there is generally a central corneal opacification, sometimes associated with microphthalmia. Such a presentation in the presence of a prominent forehead, long philtrum, and dysplastic ears may be the manifestations of Peter's plus syndrome, in which short stature and mental retardation may be expected to emerge with time. More commonly, think of unusual presentations of **Marfan syndrome** in such patients and examine for arachnodactyly, excess joint laxity, and a family history suggestive of dissecting aneurysm. Likewise, be aware of the association with aniridia and the possibility of a chromosome 11p–related predisposition to **Wilms tumour-Aniridia-Genital anomaly-Retardation syndrome** (WAGR), in which ptosis and genital anomalies are common.

Investigations to Consider As a nonspecific finding in many karyotypic abnormalities, in the absence of a specific diagnosis from ophthalmic examination, chromosomal evaluation is indicated. 11p deletion and 20p deletion are described in WAGR and Alagille syndromes, respectively, but are not consistent reliable findings. Radiologic demonstration of butterfly vertebrae is valuable in securing an Alagille diagnosis. Mutation analysis for Fibrillin1 (*FBNI*) may be useful should a Marfan syndrome diagnosis seem likely but insecure clinically, while *PAX6* mutations are reported in some familial cases of ectopic pupils.

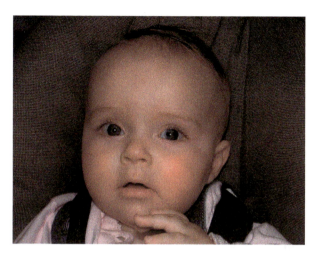

Figure 3.9 The clinical presentation of left-sided ectopic pupil is shown in a developmentally normal 9-month-old child. The family history of glaucoma in her father and grandaunt suggested a diagnosis of Rieger syndrome.

3.10 Blue Sclerae

Recognizing the Sign The darkly pigmented choroid layer often confers a rather blue appearance to the naturally thin sclera of the neonate. As a denser connective tissue construction to the sclera develops during the first several months of life, this natural phenomenon of transient blueness of the neonatal sclera disappears, usually by the age of 1 year. Persistence of the clinical sign beyond this age may be diagnostically significant and, obviously, blue sclera in a younger child may be diagnostically important and not just a transient phenomenon.

Establishing a Differential Diagnosis Most clinicians will be aware of the association between blue sclera and **osteogenesis imperfecta** (OI) and will seek a history of fractures and delayed tooth eruption and examine for bony deformation, signs of scoliosis, and joint hyperextensibility. Useful clues may be derived from the family history, particularly in cases where multiple fractures are not a major clinical problem and the diagnosis may have been hitherto unsuspected. However, blue sclera should also prompt examination for other **connective tissue diseases**, specifically Marfan syndrome and Ehlers-Danlos syndrome (EDS). In the case of **Marfan syndrome,** observe for the tall, slim appearance; joint hyperextensibility; arachnodactyly; and sternal malformations, either carinatum or excavatum. Parental height and family history, particularly with a view to sudden unexplained death in early adult life, may offer corroborative evidence. Many of these features will overlap with the **Ehlers-Danlos syndrome** complex of phenotypes, but the family history and clinical demonstration of skin hyperextensibility, excessive scarring in response to a relatively trivial injury, and easy bruising will alert the wary to a diagnosis of EDS type I. Blue sclera, skin scarring, and extreme joint laxity will not distinguish between EDS types I and EDS type VI, an autosomal recessive condition, but scoliosis and multiple criss-cross lines on the palms and soles are redolent of EDS type VI, in which eye examination is important because of associated glaucoma and propensity to rupture of the globe. Blue sclera in a small baby, particularly if the growth concerns predate birth, may be the signal to **Russell-Silver syndrome**. The examination should focus on seeking other clues such as skeletal asymmetry, relative macrocephaly, café-au-lait patches, and a clammy sweatiness, best identified by direct questioning of the mother.

Investigations to Consider X-ray evaluation looking for evidence of healed fractures, bony deformities, and wormian bones in the cranial sutures is the mainstay of diagnosis in OI. If clinical doubt exists, mutation analysis of the *FBNI* gene may be undertaken in Marfan syndrome, while lysyl hydroxylase deficiency in cultured skin fibroblasts is demonstrable in many cases of EDS type VI. A good screening test is urinary pyridinoline cross-linkages.

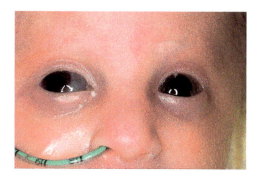

Figure 3.10 Blue sclera in a severe case of osteogenesis imperfecta.

3.11 Iris Coloboma

Recognizing the Sign The term coloboma signifies a fissure in the iris. Since the iris derives embryologically from the neural retina and the pigment epithelium of the optic cup, the clinical significance of an iris coloboma is that it may be the visible sign of an embryologically associated underlying coloboma of the retina.

Establishing a Differential Diagnosis Ophthalmologic examination is crucial not only to establish the extent of embryologic defect, but also to identify any associated abnormalities such as cataract or retinal detachment. In terms of the general clinical examination of the baby with iris colobomata, specific evaluation for clinical signs of **CHARGE association** (*c*oloboma, *h*eart defects, *a*tresia choana, *r*etardation of growth and development, *g*enital anomaly, and *e*ar malformation) is important. Frequently, the external ear is the most noteworthy sign, often comprising a simple, cup-shaped or, less commonly, an overfolded helix. Iris coloboma and dysplastic ears will also be encountered in **Catel-Manzke syndrome,** but the cleft palate and bizarrely deviated index finger will betray this specific diagnosis. The presence of preauricular pits or tags will alert the clinician to the possible diagnosis of **cat-eye syndrome,** and examination should specifically be extended to assess for anal stenosis and possible evidence, depending on age at examination, of developmental delay (Figure 4.8). The observation of hypertelorism in association with iris coloboma should prompt evaluation for **Wolf-Hirschhorn syndrome**, looking specifically at the glabellar region for prominence and at the nose for the Greek helmet profile (Figure 2.3A). Microcephaly, cleft lip, or a midline scalp defect would strongly support such diagnostic thoughts. By contrast, **Gorlin syndrome**, in which iris coloboma is seen in the context of macrocephaly and there is a propensity to basal cell carcinoma of the skin, is rarely diagnosable by examination of the newborn in isolation, but the family history in this autosomal dominant condition will explain the significance of the iris coloboma, and the later emergence of the nevoid basal cell carcinomas should be anticipated. A rare but important association is **neurofibromatosis type I** (NF1), signifying the need for longitudinal follow-up lest café-au-lait and other characteristic signs emerge.

Investigations to Consider Cardiac evaluation is mandatory if CHARGE, cat-eye, or Wolf-Hirschhorn syndromes are suspected. Computed tomography (CT) scan of the petrous temporal bone in CHARGE shows hypoplasia of the semicircular canals. FISH is indicated for 4p deletion in Wolf-Hirschhorn syndrome, while karyotype in cat-eye syndrome usually shows additional chromosome 22 material. Occasionally, FISH needs to be undertaken to establish the cause of the clinical signs. X-ray in Catel-Manzke will show an accessory phalanx at the base of the index finger.

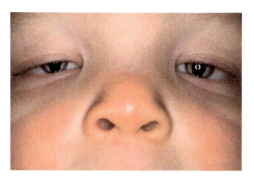

Figure 3.11 Bilateral iris colobomata are demonstrated in this patient.

3.12 Anophthalmia/Microphthalmia

Recognizing the Sign Anophthalmia signifies complete absence of outgrowth from the optic vesicle and failure of the eye to form. This very rarely occurs and the more likely situation clinically is of "cryptophthalmos," where a fusion of the eyelid obscures the orbit beneath, which may itself be abnormal, perhaps colobomatous, or microphthalmic. Microphthalmia refers to an abnormally small eye, often seen in conjunction with narrow palpebral fissures and deep-set eyes. Obviously, full ophthalmic characterization of the lesions is important.

Establishing a Differential Diagnosis The history, particularly of antenatal exposure or intrauterine infection, may be significant, **TORCH** agents, **alcohol,** and **warfarin** all being established causes of microphthalmia. Likewise, pure familial forms are well reported, so the family history may give a clue. In the established absence of such issues, examine the ears for signs of **CHARGE association** and consider evidence for choanal atresia/stenosis in the form of mouth breathing or persistent runny nose. Simple ear helices, cleft lip, or sloping shoulders due to hypoplasia of the lateral element of the clavicles are the clinical clues to **Lenz microphthalmia syndrome**. Microcephaly is usual and will be associated with developmental delay. Being X-linked, this is an important diagnosis to secure. The same applies to **Lowe syndrome**, again inherited as an X-linked disorder, in which the deep-set, microphthalmic eyes of the neonate may be the clue to diagnosis. In **oculo-dento-digital syndrome**, the microphthalmia will generally be associated with hypotelorism and skin syndactyly, typically of fingers 3 to 5 (Figure 2.2). Syndactyly of a more general nature is characteristic of **Fraser syndrome**, in which cryptophthalmia is generally observed, often with a protrusion of the anterior hairline toward the orbital margin. Look for genital malformations, typically hypospadias or clitoromegaly, and low-set ears for corroborative evidence of this autosomal recessive condition. Finally, examine the skin carefully, as linear areas of dermal hypoplasia, perhaps erythematous in the neonate and pigmented or atrophic in the older child are likely to signify the diagnosis of **Goltz syndrome** (focal dermal hypoplasia).

Investigations to Consider Aminoaciduria is usual in Lowe syndrome, though it may be normal neonatally. Urinary retinol binding protein may be a better assay for screening. Ophthalmic examination of carrier females for visually insignificant cortical opacities is valuable, almost all carriers showing this sign. Ultrasound of the kidneys may show renal agenesis in Fraser syndrome. Mutation analysis of the *BCOR* gene on Xq27 is required to confirm Lenz syndrome. Chromosomal evaluation has shown Xp22 microdeletions in a handful of cases of linear skin lesions with microphthalmia.

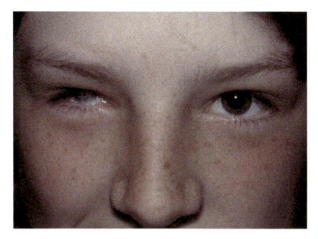

Figure 3.12 Note the discrepancy in size between the eyes. The microphthalmic eye is deep set and shows sclerocornea. (Courtesy of Mr. D. Brosnihan.)

3.13 Iris Variants

Recognizing the Sign Within the normal population, the iris demonstrates variation in color and pattern. However, there are some well-delineated, syndromically important, specific iris patterns: (1) Brushfield spots are white or yellowish speckled dots on the iris, usually toward the periphery; (2) stellate iris, meaning a lacy pattern, sometimes described as resembling the outward radiation of the spokes of a bicycle wheel; (3) cloverleaf iris (also known as Lester's sign), in which a collarette of dark pigmentation around the central part of the iris is surrounded by lighter pigment; (4) Lisch nodules, which are hamartomatous in nature and clinically present brown or cream colored well-defined elevations, randomly distributed on the surface of the iris, and generally visible on close inspection, though confirmation of whose absence necessitates slit lamp examination; and (5) heterochromia iridum in which the color of one iris differs from the other (but the term is also used to denote color variation within the same iris).

Establishing a Differential Diagnosis Brushfield spots are invariably linked in the clinical mind to **Down syndrome,** and associated signs of macroglossia, brachycephaly, single palmar creases, and clinodactyly will automatically be assessed. Remember that these iris pigmentary phenomena are also seen in 10% of normal neonates. Beware of potential confusion with Zellweger syndrome, in which hepatomegaly and extreme hypotonia also occur. The stellate iris is also a phenomenon of 10% of the normal population, but noted in up to 75% of blue-eyed **Williams syndrome** cases. Examine for the supra-valvular aortic stenosis and other cardiac signs and look clinically for the wide mouth and long, usually smooth philtrum. Lester's sign is seen in 50% of cases of **nail-patella syndrome**, in which absent or hypoplastic nails affect the thumb most commonly (Figure 12.1). Small patellae, tending to recurrent subluxation, are a feature of older children. Lisch nodules betoken **neurofibromatosis type 1** (NF1) and a search for other clinical signs, such as café-au-lait patches, freckling, and neurofibromata, is indicated. Do check for optic glioma, scoliosis, and hypertension. Heterochromia iridium should prompt evaluation of other hypopigmentation signs, such as premature greying in the family, assessment of hearing, and specific examination for telecanthus, all characteristic of **Waardenburg syndrome**.

Investigations to Consider Karyotype will confirm Down syndrome. FISH for *ELN* on chromosome 7q is required for Williams syndrome confirmation. Very-long-chain fatty acids are generally abnormal in Zellweger cases, and Waardenburg syndrome diagnosis is confirmed by *PAX3* mutation analysis if dystopia canthorum is present (type I) and *MITF* mutation analysis if absent (type II) (Figure 12.7A).

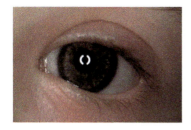

Figure 3.13A Brushfield spots.

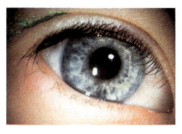

Figure 13.3B Stellate iris.

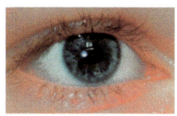

Figure 13.3C Lester' sign. (Courtesy of Dr. Elizabeth Sweeney.)

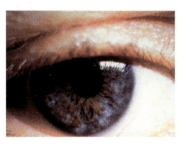

Figure 13.3D Lisch nodule.

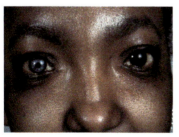

Figure 13.3E Heterochromia iridum.

3.14 Ectropion of the Lower Eyelid

Recognizing the Sign The normal position of the lower eyelid is such that it sits against the globe. Ectropion is present when the lower eyelid, through excess tissue or loss of elasticity, no longer approximates to the globe and a gap is visible between the eyelid margin and the globe. There may be eversion of the eyelid margin, whose capillary bed becomes visible.

Establishing a Differential Diagnosis Particular attention to the examination of the skin is advised. In a newborn, ectropion accompanies **lamellar ichthyosis** (collodion baby syndrome; Figure 12.15). The skin looks shiny and cracks, peeling away to reveal normal skin beneath over a period of a few weeks. The ectropion usually resolves. Persisting ectropion may betoken **cutis laxa syndrome**. Look for redundant folds of excess skin, often best observed over the neck, the dorsum of the hands, and the chest. Tachypnea is an important clue, as many of these patients develop early-onset emphysema and succumb to cor pulmonale. Other valuable clinical clues are scars of surgical treatment for umbilical or inguinal herniae. The presence of a cleft lip and/or palate is likely to signify the autosomal dominant condition of **blepharo-cheilo-dontic (BCD) syndrome**, and parental examination for oligodontia, ectropion, and double row of eyelashes (distichiasis) may secure this diagnosis in the parent and child. Cardiac abnormalities should be sought if the diagnosis is **Kabuki syndrome**, in which the facial characteristics are of wide palpebral fissures and ectropion. Mild developmental delay is usual. Specifically helpful clinical features are persisting fetal finger pads (Figure 9.16) and eyebrows that may be excessively arched and are often deficient of hair in the middle. A history of early feeding difficulty, perhaps requiring nasogastric supplementation, is common. The author has twice been prompted to this diagnosis by persisting blue sclerae in children aged 2 years. Family history of parathyroid, medullary thyroid, or pheochromocytoma in a child with ectropion is almost certain to represent **multiple endocrine neoplasia type IIB** (MEN IIB). The lips may be thickened and nodular and the tongue likewise. Malar hypoplasia, downslanting palpebral fissures, and ectropion, the facial features of **Miller syndrome**, should prompt examination of the hands, the little fingers and toes usually being absent.

Investigations to Consider Clinical examination is often adequate to secure the diagnosis. Bladder diverticula may be radiologically demonstrable in cutis laxa. *RET* gene mutations are demonstrable in MEN IIB.

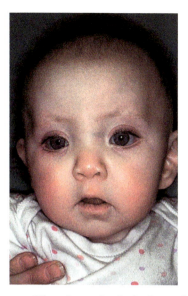

Figure 3.14 Bilateral ectropion is clearly seen in this patient with Kabuki syndrome. Additional dysmorphic features associated with Kabuki syndrome to observe are the wide palpebral fissures, blue sclerae, and relative thinning of eyebrow hair in the midzone of the eyebrows ("interrupted eyebrows"). There is also a lower lip pit, a common observation in cases of Kabuki syndrome.

3.15 Eyebrow Variants

Recognizing the Sign It is worth evaluating the eyebrows in terms of their position and shape and confirming that they are present. Diagnostically useful variants to observe are (1) sparse/absent eyebrows; (2) arched eyebrows, in which the natural arch of the eyebrow configuration is exaggerated; (3) laterally deficient or luxuriant eyebrows; and (4) medially flared eyebrows.

Establishing a Differential Diagnosis Absent eyebrows should direct clinical attention to ectodermally derived tissues, the skin, the nails, and the hair for possible signs of **ectodermal dysplasia**. Fine scalp hair, absent sweating, and a history of recurrent fever episodes probably signify the X-linked form, and hypodontia or anodontia in other family members is corroborative. Periorbital hyperpigmentation and a slightly dry, wrinkled texture to the skin around the eyes are good clues, as is family history. In the presence of cleft lip or palate, eyebrow absence prompts the diagnosis of **Rapp-Hodgkin syndrome**. Coarse, slow-growing hair is typical, and a family history of early hair loss in this autosomal dominant condition is diagnostically significant. Hypospadias is common in affected males. Exaggerated arching of the eyebrows is one of the diagnostic hallmarks of **Kabuki syndrome** noted by the original authors, but relative deficiency of hair growth in the mid-eyebrow region is probably more common ("interrupted eyebrow sign"). Ectropion, fetal finger pads, and cardiac defects should be sought. Luxuriance of the lateral aspect of the eyebrow is described in **Noonan syndrome**, but is only corroborative if major signs of that condition, such as ptosis, low posterior hairline, or cardiac malformations, have already prompted the diagnosis (Figure 6.1). By contrast, medial thickening of the eyebrow can be a good prompt to the diagnosis of **tricho-rhino-phalangeal (TRP) syndrome** and directs the examiner toward the nose for the bulbous nasal tip redolent of this condition (Figure 2.4A). Likewise, unusual angulation of the digits at the interphalangeal joints is worthy of the examiner's attention in cases of TRP. Medial eyebrow flaring is also a feature of **Williams syndrome**, so evaluation for the stellate iris pattern, the characteristic lip fullness, and evidence of cardiac murmur is sensible. Finally, consider **Waardenburg syndrome**, the medical eyebrow flare sometimes resulting in synophrys. Deafness and features of hypopigmentation in the skin and hair should be sought.

Investigations to Consider Mutation analysis of the *EDA1* gene on Xq12 confirms X-linked hypohidrotic dysplasia if there is clinical doubt. TRP syndrome cases should have chromosome 8q24 deletion studies, especially if the patient shows developmental delay. FISH for *ELN* will confirm Williams syndrome. *PAX3, MITF,* and *SOX10* mutations can generate a Waardenburg phenotype.

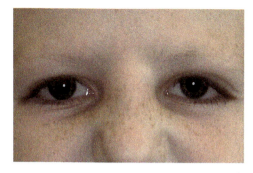

Figure 3.15A Sparse eyebrows.

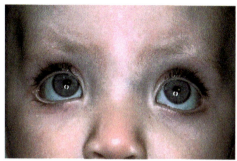

Figure 3.15B Interrupted eyebrow, lower lid ectropion, and wide palpebral fissure in Kabuki syndrome.

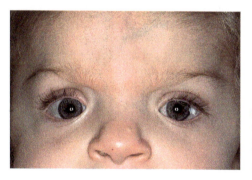

Figure 3.15C Medial flare of the eyebrow and dystopia canthorum in Waardenburg syndrome type I.

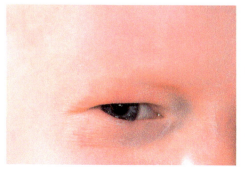

Figure 3.5D Absence of the eyebrows is demonstrated in a patient with X-linked hypohydrotic ectodermal dysplasia syndrome. Note the very characteristic fine periorbital wrinkling.

3.16   Eyelash Variants

Recognizing the Sign   The normal configuration of the eyelashes follows a gentle outward curve from the eyelid, with the upper and lower lashes meeting but not interdigitating on lid closure.

Establishing a Differential Diagnosis   Straight eyelashes in a neonate who is feeding poorly are a feature of **myopathic conditions** and are observed in situations that can present as a myopathy, such as Prader-Willi syndrome. This diagnosis is not made on the configuration of the eyelash alone, but the clinical observation can drive the investigation in a particular direction. Generalized hirsutism is frequently associated with long, perhaps eccentrically oriented, eyelashes. Look over the back for hair whorls. Think specifically of **de Lange syndrome** and assess for microcephaly and generalized increased tone and examine the hands for malformations and specifically for proximally placed thumbs due to the characteristically short first metacarpal (Figure 9.13B). Long eyelashes in a patient in whom you think there is floppiness or evidence of delayed motor milestones might prompt you to look for retinal pigmentary disorders, as these features comprise a rare autosomal recessive mental retardation disorder associated with variously disordered pituitary malfunction, **chorioretinitis-pituitary dysfunction syndrome**. A family history of lymphoedema from around the age of puberty should prompt examination for **distichiasis**, a double row of eyelashes, which can scratch the conjunctiva and be a severe irritant to patients. The condition of **lymphoedema-distichiasis syndrome** is autosomal dominant, and congenital heart disease should be sought. Absence of eyelashes is frequently observed in **ectodermal dysplasias**, in consequence of which a careful evaluation of the skin, nails, hair, and dentition as well as family history may give clues to the underlying diagnosis. Absent eyelashes, especially if there are dermatologic signs such as palmoplantar skin thickening, knuckle thickening, or leukonychia (white nails), should prompt assessment of hearing, as there are a range of deafness syndromes associated. Short limbs in a baby with sparse hair and eyebrow and eyelash absence may be the clues to **McKusick-Cartilage-Hair hypoplasia syndrome**, an important autosomal recessive condition to recognize because of the associated immunodeficiency and particular susceptibility to varicella infection, often with fatal outcome.

Investigations to Consider   Paternal deletion of chromosome 15q is demonstrable either cytogenetically or by DNA analysis in most cases of Prader-Willi syndrome. If deafness is suspected, connexin 26 and 30 (*GJB2 and GJB6*) mutation should be sought. Radiologic characteristics of cartilage hair hypoplasia apart from short, wide bones are metaphyseal dysplasia, particularly of the lower end of the femur, and cone-shaped epiphyses of the phalanges.

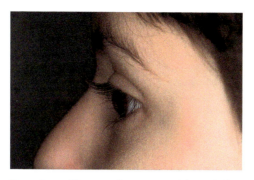

Figure 3.16A The normal curvature of the eyelashes is shown.

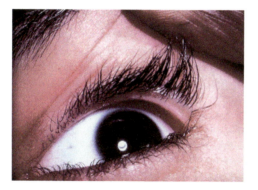

Figure 3.16B A double row of eyelashes is shown in a patient with lymphoedema-distichiasis syndrome. Note the bizarre course of some of the hairs that are directed toward the cornea and frequently cause corneal irritation and abrasion. (Courtesy of Mr. D. Brosnihan.)

3.17 Epibulbar Dermoid

Recognizing the Sign These are solid tumors of the ocular surface, usually a pearly grey color, comprising collagen with an epidermal covering or, occasionally, adipose tissue. They may be unilateral or bilateral and are most likely to be noticed if at the limbus. However, most occur on the bulbar conjunctiva and as such, may be identified only by retraction of the eyelid for examination.

Establishing a Differential Diagnosis Examine the eye thoroughly. Note whether the iris looks normal, whether the pupil is central, and whether there is any evidence of corneal opacity, and seek evidence of other dermoid tumors on the conjunctiva. Look at the eyelids for coloboma. Pediatric ophthalmologic evaluation is indicated to assess normality of ocular structures. Assess the face for evidence of asymmetry and the ears for preauricular tags and/or microtia. The presence of epibulbar dermoid and asymmetric facial weakness suggests a likely diagnosis of **Goldenhar syndrome** spectrum, in which condition examination for congenital heart disease should form part of the assessment, as should examination of hearing. Awareness of the high likelihood of associated cervical hemivertebra is important to investigation and future management. Isolated corneal dermoids are described in autosomal dominant, recessive, and X-linked pedigrees, for which reason family history and parental examination can be useful. Careful examination of the skin is important in isolated cases of epibulbar dermoid lest this be the presenting feature of **linear sebaceous nevus syndrome**. The signs in this condition can be protean, but look out for slightly elevated, yellow or tan skin plaques, which often acquire a verrucous appearance with time. The association of the condition with progressive macrocephaly, cranial nerve palsy, mental retardation, and bone cysts should be borne in mind. Deafness concerns in a child with epibulbar dermoid are not confined to the Goldenhar spectrum, but a history of anal stenosis suggests **Townes-Brocks syndrome** (TBS). Look carefully at the thumbs, where the terminal phalanx is often at an odd angle with respect to the proximal phalanx, due to the presence of an accessory phalanx (Figure 9.14D). Likewise, the anus may be anteriorly placed. Many of these features, including preauricular pits, congenital heart disease, and anal stenosis, overlap with marker chromosome 22 syndrome (Figure 4.8).

Investigations to Consider Neck radiology is indicated if Goldenhar syndrome seems likely. Chromosomal studies, if necessary of the fibroblasts, should be undertaken if marker 22 is suspected. Mutation of *SAL1* is demonstrable in most patients with TBS and even a few cases that clinically overlap with Goldenhar syndrome.

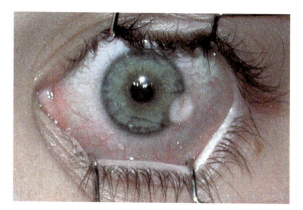

Figure 3.17 Note the grey colored dermoid demonstrated at the limbus.

Chapter 4　**The Ear**

4.1 Low-Set Ears

Recognizing the Sign Low-set ears are one of the most commonly attributed and least specific of clinical signs in dysmorphology, and an endless source of confused argument. The definition of the sign is governed by the drawing of an imaginary horizontal line through the outer canthi of the eyes, and the ears are adjudged to be low set if the root of the helix falls below this line (Figure 4.1A).

Establishing a Differential Diagnosis Bear in mind that hydrocephalus, macrocephaly, and unusually small but normally shaped ears distort the normal relative proportions between these anatomic features, resulting in low-set ears. In view of the nonspecificity of the clinical sign, the purpose of clinical examination is to establish the presence of other anomalies that may facilitate the emergence of an underlying diagnosis. Observe whether the ear is normal or has other anomalous features, such as of helical shape, which are dealt with in later sections of this chapter. Relatively common genetic syndromes in which low-set ears are frequently encountered include **Noonan syndrome** and **velo-cardio-facial (VCF) syndrome**. The associated features in Noonan syndrome of family history of short stature, ptosis, heart murmur, typically pulmonary stenosis, low posterior hairline, and excess nuchal skin will betray the true diagnosis. VCF syndrome is more variable, but the presence of a heart murmur; suspected palatal incompetence or cleft; feeding problems, especially nasal regurgitation of milk; hypocalcemia; or facial palsy may all serve to prompt the diagnosis. The identification of hypospadias in a patient with low-set ears should raise the possibility that the patient has **Smith-Lemli-Opitz syndrome** (S-L-O), further substantiated if 2/3 toe syndactyly, ptosis, and microcephaly and developmental concerns complete the clinical presentation. Microcephaly and low-set ears are also common in **Rubinstein-Taybi syndrome**, but the characteristic nasal configuration, the septum extending below the ala nasi, and the broad thumbs will clearly signal this diagnosis in all but the most subtle of cases. The finding of joint dislocations and/or restricted joint movement with low-set ears may be the clues to the autosomal recessive condition of **Pena-Shokeir syndrome**; early diagnosis is important as neonatal death frequently follows from associated pulmonary hypoplasia.

Investigations to Consider The identification of associated clinical findings, unless syndrome specific, merit karyotype investigation. Fluorescence in situ hybridization (FISH) of 22q11 will confirm or refute concerns for VCF syndrome. S-L-O patients have low plasma cholesterol but raised 7-dehydrocholesterol. Identification of the associated coagulopathy is valuable if Noonan syndrome cases are undergoing surgery. Only a minority of Rubinstein-Taybi (R-T) cases show a chromosome 15 deletion by FISH, and if confirmation of diagnosis is required, molecular analysis must be resorted to.

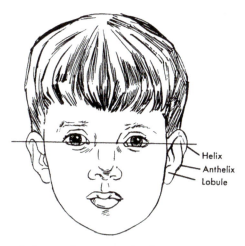

Figure 4.1A A scematic representation demonstrating ear place-ment relative to a horizontal line through the outer canthi of the eyes. The ears are considered low-set when the root of the helix is below this line. (With acknowledgment to Stevenson and Hall, *Human Malformations and Related Anomalies*, second edition. Oxford University Press, 2006.)

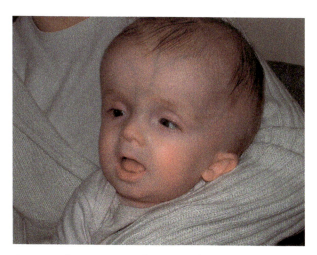

Figure 4.1B Low-set ears are demonstrated as a secondary phe-nomenon in a boy with hydrocephalus.

4.2 Posteriorly Rotated Ears

Recognizing the Sign This term describes the position of the external ear whose vertical axis has been rotated posteriorly. It therefore follows that a posteriorly rotated ear is likely to be low set, and in fact, posterior rotation is the most common cause of a seemingly low-set ear.

Establishing a Differential Diagnosis Posteriorly rotated ears are a common, nonspecific finding on clinical examination and their significance has to be weighted with respect to other clinical findings. However, be aware of the posteriorly rotated ears as an easy clue to **Noonan syndrome** and look out for ptosis, excess nuchal skin, and other corroborative signs. There are two closely overlapping syndromes to bear in mind: cardio-facio-cutaneous (CFC) syndrome and Costello syndrome. **CFC syndrome** should be considered in a Noonan-like child, usually with pulmonary stenosis or an atrial septal defect (ASD) but in whom the hair growth is poor and the skin dry, usually itchy and even ichthyotic. Loose skin on the hands and feet and unexplained liver enlargement are other clinical findings of diagnostic value. **Costello syndrome** shares the features of excess loose skin on the palms and soles, often with areas of extreme hyperkeratosis on pressure areas. Characteristically, nasal papillomata develop around the age of 6. Developmental delay is the norm in Costello cases, and an additional finding is the ulnar deviation of the rest position of the hands. Examination of the skin is also important in suspecting the diagnosis of **carbohydrate-deficient glycoprotein (CDG) syndrome**, with unusual distribution of fat pads around the pubis or buttocks being important to assess. Inversion of the nipples against a background history of probable developmental delay in a nondysmorphic child, often with posterior rotation of the ears, may be a valuable prompt to this diagnosis. By contrast, an extra nipple should prompt consideration of **Simpson-Golabi-Behmel (SGB) syndrome**, and inquiry for high birth weight and examination of the tongue for a deep midline groove, the heart for murmur, and the hands for evidence of surgically removed polydactyly and small nails on the index fingers are the way to proceed. Large, posteriorly rotated ears in a baby who is failing to thrive may signify **Richardson-Kirk syndrome**, an autosomal recessive disorder with hypoparathyroidism and immunocompromise. Check the fontanelle for delayed closure.

Investigations to Consider Echocardiography should be undertaken if Noonan, CFC, Costello, or SGB syndromes are clinically suspected. Mutation analysis of *GPC3* on Xq27 will confirm diagnosis in SGB. Radiology of the long bones usually shows medullary stenosis and cortical thickening in Richardson-Kirk. Hypoparathyroidism should be sought biochemically. Mutation analysis of the *TBCE* gene on chromosome 1 is confirmatory.

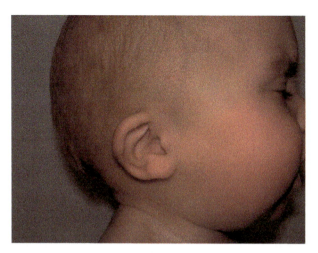

Figure 4.2 Posterior rotation of the ear is demonstrated in a boy with cardiofaciocutaneous syndrome. Other clues to this diagnosis in his case are shown—note the sparse scalp hair, the rash, the thick bushy eyebrows, the long and somewhat chaotic eyelashes, and his high cheek color.

4.3 Auricular Pits

Recognizing the Sign These commonly observed clinical features comprise blind-ending, shallow invaginations whose entrance is typically seen just anterior to the insertion of the helix of the ear. Bilateral in approximately 20% of cases, they also occur in front of the tragus of the ear, sometimes associated with preauricular appendages. Pits on the helical rim are rare and are specifically associated with Beckwith-Wiedemann syndrome.

Establishing a Differential Diagnosis While most preauricular pits are of no diagnostic significance, the clinical examination should specifically address the possibility that the patient may have **branchio-oto-renal (BOR) syndrome**, preauricular pits being especially redolent of that disorder. Observe the neck for sinuses and seek a family history of neck sinus surgery or use of hearing aids, which might suggest this autosomal dominant condition. Examine for deafness, typically conductive. The external ear may be misshapen and hypoplastic, while the ear canal may be narrow and upslanting. Much phenotypic overlap can exist between BOR syndrome and a genetically distinct syndrome, **Townes-Brocks Syndrome** (TBS), in which lop ears (malformation of the superior portion of the ear and associated floppiness of the helix), microtia, and ear pits are associated with deviated distal phalanges of the thumb, due to the presence of an additional phalanx (Figure 9.14D). Classically, affected individuals have anal stenosis and, even if absent, excess perianal skin, anterior placement of the anus, and midline perianal raphe extending between the scrotum and the anus are important discriminating clues to the diagnosis of TBS. Deafness should be sought by history and assessment of hearing. Ear pits along a line from the tragus to the mouth are seen in cases of **Treacher Collins syndrome**, but the narrow face of the hypoplastic zygomas and lower eyelid colobomata will allow distinction of this cause of pits from other syndromes. The facial asymmetry, often with asymmetric microtia and, possibly, epibulbar dermoid of **Goldenhar syndrome,** is certainly associated with auricular pits in a minority of instances. Examine behind the ear for hemangioma, which signals the rare autosomal dominant condition **branchio-oculo-facial (BOF) syndrome** and for colobomata of the eye, lip pits, and very prominent philtral pillars giving an impression of treated cleft lip, which are additional valuable signs.

Investigations to Consider Renal ultrasound for renal aplasia, hypoplasia, and collecting system malformations is indicated in BOR syndrome and TBS. Biochemical indices of renal function are indicated in BOR syndrome and TBS. Hand radiology in TBS assesses for possible triphalangeal thumbs. Computed tomography (CT) scan of the petrous temporal bone in BOR syndrome usually shows middle ear flattening and ossicular malformations. Mutation of *SALL1* confirms TBS, while *EYA1* is the main locus for BOR syndrome.

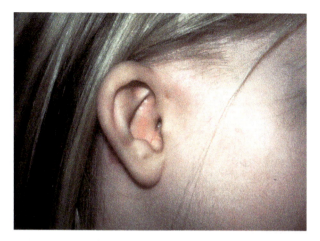

Figure 4.3A Typical preauricular position of the pit in a patient with branchio-oto-renal syndrome. Though slightly cupped, the external ear is essentially normal. (See also Figure 4.4.)

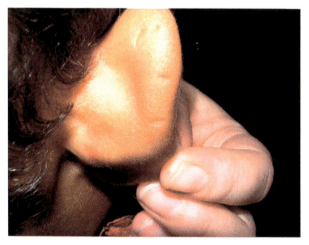

Figure 4.3B Several discrete depressions are visible on the posterior surface of the helical rim in a case of Beckwith-Wiedemann syndrome. (See also Figure 4.4.)

4.4 Microtia

Recognizing the Sign Microtia is a widely embracing term signifying a spectrum of external ear malformations from a structurally normal but small ear to complete absence of auricular structures, most commonly represented by some identifiable cartilaginous presence, often with preauricular tags or accessory auricles.

Establishing a Differential Diagnosis Observe whether the external auditory canal is atretic or patent. Atresia is common in cases of microtia and conductive hearing disruption attends, irrespective of any associated underlying cochlear malformation. Look at the face, specifically for facial asymmetry and/or facial nerve palsy, both of which suggest a possible underlying diagnosis of **Goldenhar syndrome** (oculoauriculovertebral). Examine the eye for an epibulbar dermoid, which confirms Goldenhar syndrome. A prenatal history of **maternal diabetes or alcohol** exposure is significant, microtia being described in both situations. Assess for other clinical features of embryopathy, congenital heart defects, and preaxial polydactyly of the feet in diabetes, and microcephaly, short palpebral fissures, smooth philtrum, and mild degrees of finger syndactyly in alcohol exposure. Both **Nager and Miller syndromes** are associated with microtia, the underlying diagnosis being identifiable by the limb abnormalities. The facial features in both these conditions are reminiscent of Treacher Collins syndrome, with malar hypoplasia, downslanting palpebral fissures, sometimes lower eyelid colobomata, and micrognathia, but the distinction in limb malformations affords diagnostic accuracy—absence or hypoplasia of the thumbs and/or radii characterizes Nager syndrome, and Miller syndrome typically has fifth digit absence. Abnormal angulation of the thumbs in a child with microtia probably betrays a diagnosis of **Townes-Brocks syndrome** (Figure 9.14D) and anterior placement of the anus, or a history of anal stenosis would be entirely consistent. Likewise, microtia can be seen in **branchio-oto-renal** (BOR) **syndrome**, the family history of or recognition on clinical examination of branchial sinuses being specific clues (Figure 4.5A). The presence of an iris coloboma should alert the clinician to the possibility that the underlying condition is **CHARGE association** (*c*oloboma, *h*eart, *a*tresia choana, *r*etarded growth, *g*enital abnormalities, *e*ar malformations), but the ear anomalies are generally at the mild end of microtia, with a recognizable external ear of unusual shape rather than a misshapen cartilaginous rudiment.

Investigations to Consider Audiologic evaluation is essential. Conductive loss is common, associated with ossicular malformation. Sensorineural loss is rarer, generally with underlying cochlear malformation, for which reason CT scan of the petrous temporal bone to assess both middle ear and cochlear morphology is indicated. Neck radiology should be undertaken to assess possible cervical vertebral fusion if facial asymmetry is seen. Cardiac echography is indicated in cases of possible CHARGE, and renal investigations if BOR syndrome is suspected.

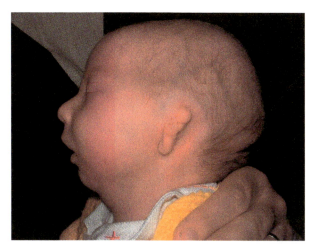

Figure 4.4 Severe microtia in a case of Treacher Collins syndrome. Several auricular pits are visible on the malformed ear in this patient, who also has a pit on the cheek, which is often seen in Treacher Collins cases.

4.5 External Ear Variants

Recognizing the Sign The architecture of the external ear is subject to significant variability within the normal range. Some specific configurations do have particular diagnostic and pathologic implications, though it should be established that most of these clinical signs are usually isolated and of no underlying significance: (1) "lop ear," a term of wide embrace but which broadly refers to a loss of normal shape of the superior part of the helix, which then cups anteriorly; (2) crumpled ears, in which additional extra folds in the cartilage confer a crumpled appearance on the auricle; (3) protruding ears ("bat ears"), in which the whole ear stands out prominently from the side of the head, the distance from the outer rim of the helix to the mastoid being greater than 2 cm; and (4) cryptotia, in which the superior helical rim is less well demarcated from adjacent scalp skin than usual, appearing to be continuous with the lateral scalp.

Establishing a Differential Diagnosis Lop ears should prompt examination for other possible features of **branchio-oto-renal (BOR) syndrome** and **Townes-Brocks** (TBS) syndrome. Long, abnormal angulation of the thumbs suggests TBS, as does anal stenosis or anterior placement of the anus, while branchial sinuses or a family history of such betray BOR. Specifically think of **CHARGE** association (Coloboma—Heart defects—Atresia choani—Retardation—Genital anomalies—Ear malformations), of which lop ear is a particular but inconstant hallmark. The observation of crumpled ears should prompt immediate thoughts of **Beals syndrome** and be followed by examination of the joints for contractures, typically of the fingers but, less commonly, of the knees, elbows, and hips. There may be arachnodactyly and the habitus is thin and marfanoid. In the older child, remember to examine for scoliosis and beware of the absence of contractures that may have responded to physiotherapy; the history, prompted by the ear configuration, will betray the diagnosis. Protruding ears are a normal variant in the population, but in the presence of neonatal hypocalcemia may be the clue to **Richardson-Kirk syndrome**, or in a male with short stature, to **Aarskog syndrome**, in which condition the shawl scrotum and hypertelorism should be sought. Cryptotia is uncommon but is seen in some cases of **Edwards syndrome** and **Fraser syndrome**, in which the anterior hairline is often irregularly low and the main clinical focus will be on the eyes, which are cryptophthalmic or microphthalmic.

Investigations to Consider Renal tract evaluation in possible BOR and TBS cases as well as biochemical indices of kidney function. Cardiac evaluation is necessary in CHARGE and Beals, specifically for mitral prolapse in the latter.

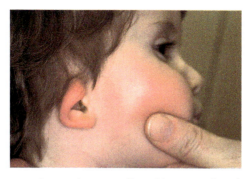

Figure 4.5A Lop ear in a case of branchio-oto-renal syndrome.

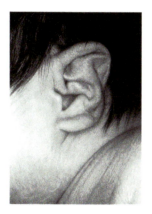

Figure 4.5B Crumpled ear.

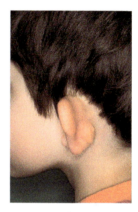

Figure 4.5C Protruding ear.

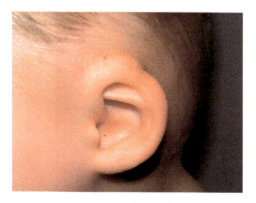

Figure 4.5D Cryptotia.

4.6 Ear Lobe Variants

Recognizing the Sign Normal variation accommodates a wide range of configurations, but there are a few that may enjoy syndromic association and therefore are diagnostically noteworthy: (1) ear lobe creases, by which is meant linear fissures on the lobule of the ear; (2) absence of the earlobe; (3) uplifted earlobes, in which the insertion of the lobe to the facial skin is above the level of the lobe so that the lobe hangs, free of medial attachment to the face; and (4) large, prominent ear lobes, disproportionate to the rest of the external ear.

Establishing a Differential Diagnosis Familial ear lobe variation is common, so obtain a family history and observe parental ears before ascribing a diagnostic significance to ear lobe variants. Creases of the ear lobe are uncommon and generally of no pathologic significance, but are specifically associated with **Beckwith-Wiedemann syndrome** (BWS), for which reason macroglossia, visceromegaly, facial nevus flammeus, and a history of neonatal hypoglycemia should be specifically sought. The prevalence of the syndrome is higher among infants conceived by assisted means. Absence of the earlobe is most frequently seen as a familial, autosomal dominant trait, but is a useful clinical signal to possible cases of **Ehlers-Danlos syndrome (EDS) type IV**. Look for thin skin; prominence of veins, particularly over the chest and shoulders; and joint laxity, and inquire for a history of easy bruising. In the clinical context of severe microcephaly, lobeless ears are likely to indicate the autosomal recessive condition **Seckel syndrome**. Uplift of the earlobes is a striking feature of important diagnostic significance in a developmentally delayed child with constipation and/or Hirschsprung's disease, indicating a likely case of **Mowat-Wilson syndrome**. Seizures, microcephaly, a prominent philtrum, a large nose, and congenital heart disease strongly support this diagnosis. Large, prominent lobes are often seen in **Costello syndrome**, so seek a history of early feeding difficulty, examine the skin for cutis laxa and the hands for ulnar drift, and, in the older child, look for nasal papillomata. Likewise, an early history of poor feeding in a child with large earlobes could signify a diagnosis of **Kabuki syndrome**. Look carefully at the lower eyelid for ectropion, at the eyebrows for possible areas of hair thinning or discontinuity, and at the lower lip for pits. In the older child, unexplained obesity is a recurrent feature of Kabuki syndrome.

Investigations to Consider Chromosome 11p15 studies for deletion, disomy, or imprinting mutations can confirm BWS if there is clinical doubt but are complex. If EDS type IV is suspected *Col3A1* mutation analysis is useful. In Mowat-Wilson, *ZFHX1B* mutation confirms the diagnosis.

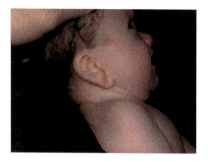

Figure 4.6A Ear lobe creases typical of Beckwith-Wiedemann syndrome.

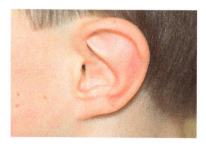

Figure 4.6B Absent ear lobes in a case of Ehlers-Danlos syndrome type IV.

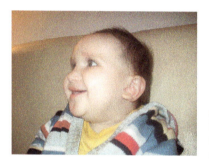

Figure 4.6C Uplifted earlobe in Mowat-Wilson syndrome. This is the same patient whose face is seen in Figure 2.5C.

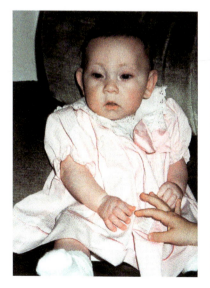

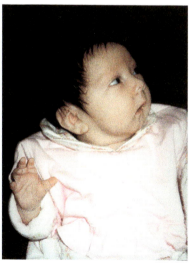

D

E

Figure 4.6D and E Prominent earlobe is demonstrated in frontal and lateral views of the same patient with Kabuki syndrome.

4.7　External Auditory Canal Atresia or Stenosis

Recognizing the Sign　Ninety percent of cases of external auditory canal atresia involve microtia and are addressed in section 4.4. The 10% of cases to which this section refers are easily missed, with the external ears being normal; the average age at diagnosis is about 3 years. The external auditory canal may be completely absent or a small external meatus may be seen, which, on otoscopy, is blind ending.

Establishing a Differential Diagnosis　Establish whether the atresia is unilateral or bilateral. The family history might be useful, rare autosomal dominant kindreds being described in which this disorder segregates. Clinical assessment of hearing should be expected to demonstrate a significant conductive hearing impairment, but there may also be a sensorineural deafness if there is associated cochlear malformation. Assess the patient's body habitus, specifically the neck for clinical suspicion of a Klippel-Feil malformation (cervical vertebral fusion). Specifically examine the external ocular movements, with particular reference to the lateral rectus. The condition known as **Wildervanck syndrome** is a rather variable syndrome combining features of Klippel-Feil malformation, sixth nerve palsy, and deafness, in a few of which cases external auditory canal atresia or extreme stenosis has been observed. In addition to assessing hearing, a general assessment of development is valuable. Early evidence of developmental delay in a baby with external auditory canal atresia should certainly prompt concerns for **chromosome 18q deletion syndrome**. Corroborative clinical findings would be microcephaly, cleft palate, nystagmus, and congenital heart defects. A carp-shaped mouth is said to be characteristic, by which term is meant a mouth downturned at the corners with a short philtrum and usually a thickened lower lip.

Investigations to Consider　Neck radiology is indicated if cervical spine malformation is suspected. CT scan of the petrous temporal bones is important, both to assess likely malformation of the middle ear chamber and ossicles and to look for cochlear malformations. Karyotype will establish gross 18q 23 deletions, but be aware that there are cases reported with a milder phenotype in terms of developmental delay in whom the external canal atresia was the clue to submicroscopic deletion of 18q23, not demonstrable by routine microscopy. The author is aware of one such individual attending normal school.

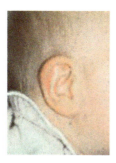

Figure 4.7 External auditory canal atresia with a normal external ear in a patient with chromosome 18q23 deletion. (Courtesy of Dr. Mohnish Suri.)

4.8 Auricular Tags

Recognizing the Sign These are easily identified and rarely confused. Fleshy, skin-covered appendages of tissue are seen, usually in front of the tragus of the ear though occasionally extending along the cheek toward the angle of the mouth, in which position it is not infrequent to observe an associated scar or pit. About 90% are unilateral.

Establishing a Differential Diagnosis Fewer than 5% are thought to represent syndromes, and most auricular tags are isolated **unilateral minor malformations of no diagnostic significance**. Opinion is divided as to the need for deafness screening in this group, but if any associated malformation of the ear is present, an underlying syndrome is more likely and such screening is certainly justified. In terms of identifying associated syndromes, microtia, facial asymmetry, epibulbar dermoid, and/or colobomata of the eyelids are strongly suggestive of **Goldenhar syndrome**, which is the most common syndrome associated with auricular tags. A history suggestive of anal stenosis may suggest **Townes-Brocks syndrome**, in which case triphalangeal thumbs should be sought. The other consideration if anal stenosis is present is **cat-eye syndrome**. This rare disorder, consequent on the presence of an additional chromosome comprising chromosome 22 material, should be suspected if there is evidence of congenital heart disease, iris coloboma, or horseshoe kidney in a child with auricular tags and/or anal stenosis.

Investigations to Consider Cervical vertebral malformation should be sought radiologically in Goldenhar cases. Mutation of *SALL1* gene confirms Townes-Brocks syndrome, while extended chromosomal analysis may be needed to adequately investigate cat-eye syndrome. Occasionally skin biopsy is required to confirm the chromosomal mosaicism, as the additional chromosome 22 material can be lost in lymphocytes.

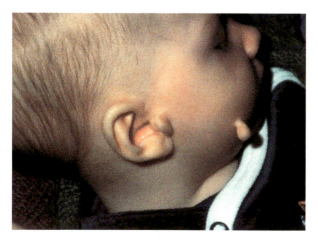

Figure 4.8A A typical example of an auricular tag, in this instance associated with a further tag on the cheek, is shown in a patient with cat-eye syndrome. Note also the preauricular pit.

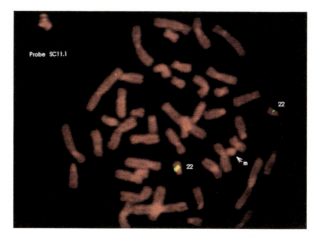

Figure 4.8B The arrow shows the marker chromosome 22 material, cytogenetically confirming the clinical diagnosis in the patient in Figure 4.8A.

Chapter 5 The Mouth and Oral Cavity

5.1 Microstomia

Recognizing the Sign Tables are available to establish whether the mouth, measured from one corner of the mouth to its opposite landmark, is enlarged or reduced outside the norm. In practice, a subjective impression is often formed looking at the face, which then informs the subsequent examination. A good rule of thumb is that the angles of the mouth are generally vertically below the pupils of the eye. Provided there are no concerns about hypotelorism, reference to the pupils can serve to confirm or refute a clinical impression of microstomia.

Establishing a Differential Diagnosis Consider the obvious by examining for micrognathia, best done in profile. Observe the symmetry of the mouth both resting and during movement and consider the associated landmarks, particularly the nasolabial folds, asymmetry of which may signify neuromuscular concerns. **Micrognathia** causing a small mouth can be identified by examination of the alveoli with the jaws held together and, instead of meeting evenly, the lower alveolar margin is well behind the upper. Asymmetric nasolabial folds at rest and asymmetric crying face on movement are occasional presenting features of both **CHARGE** (*c*oloboma, *h*eart, *a*tresia choana, *r*etarded growth, *g*enital abnormalities, *e*ar malformations) syndrome and **velo-cardio-facial (VCF) syndrome**. Hence, reference to the ears for evidence of asymmetry or microtia is sensible for CHARGE cases, as is seeking a history consistent with choanal atresia/ narrowing. Likewise, cardiac evaluation should form part of the examination in both these conditions. Carefully evaluate the hands for evidence of digital hypoplasia, seen in **hypodactyly-hypoglossia syndrome** and **Moebius syndrome**. Sixth and seventh cranial nerve palsies characterize the latter, and the pectoral muscles should be assessed for possible absence. A small tongue, perhaps anchored to the floor of the mouth, is more likely to represent hypodactyly-hypoglossia syndrome. A tightly contracted mouth usually accompanied by H-shaped puckering of the chin is the hallmark of **Freeman-Sheldon syndrome** and the diagnosis is substantiated by observing camptodactyly with ulnar deviation of the digits. Additional related clinical signs are deep-set eyes and a long philtrum. Tight contraction of the mouth in association with joint limitation and increased tone are likewise the hallmarks of **Schwartz-Jampel syndrome**, an autosomal recessive disorder that clinically overlaps with Freeman-Sheldon syndrome.

Investigations to Consider Unadorned clinical examination is the basis of several of the diagnoses discussed. Echocardiography is important if CHARGE or VCF syndromes are being considered. Fluorescence in situ hybridization (FISH) examination of 22q11 will confirm the characteristic deletion in VCF syndrome. An electromyograph may be needed to establish myotonia in Schwartz-Jampel cases. Likewise, radiologic evaluation of the vertebrae for platyspondyly and coronal clefts and of the hips for epiphyseal dysplasia is diagnostically valuable in this condition.

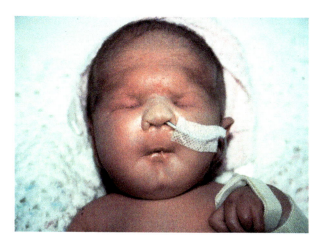

Figure 5.1 Microstomia is well demonstrated in this classical case of Freeman-Sheldon syndrome. Note additional clinical signs of the H-shaped vertical skin pucker on the chin; the deep-set, tightly closed eyes; and the camptodactyly of the fingers, showing ulnar deviation.

5.2 Upper Lip Clefts

Recognizing the Sign Embryologically, clefts derive from failure of fusion of the maxillary processes with the medial nasal processes, and clinical evidence of this failure may present with bilateral defects, unilateral defects, midline defects, a slight defect reminiscent of a scar adjacent to the margin of the philtrum (pseudocleft), or a slight dimple at the vermillion border of the lip. Some 20% of clefts are associated with an underlying syndrome.

Establishing a Differential Diagnosis Ensure that the palate is intact as cleft lip without cleft palate is empirically less likely to be associated with malformations elsewhere. The family history may offer clues consistent with autosomal dominant clefting or other important information—repair of a cleft palate in a parent should prompt examination of both parent and child for lower lip pits, which would confirm **Van der Woude syndrome**. Midline clefts, though rare, have important implications and the clinician needs to be aware of the underlying possible diagnosis of **holoprosencephaly**. Appropriate assessment for this should include evaluation for hypotelorism and optic colobomata. Parental assessment should include looking at the teeth for a single central maxillary incisor. Specific **chromosomal syndromes** to bear in mind in examining the infant presenting with cleft lip are Patau syndrome (trisomy 13), Wolf-Hirschhorn syndrome (4p16 deletion), and 1p36 deletion. A low birth weight, wide nasal bridge, and Greek helmet profile to the nose will prompt consideration of 4p deletion, especially if there is a cardiac murmur. Chromosome 1p36 deletion does not have a neonatal "gestalt" appearance, but deep-set eyes and a rather horizontal configuration to the eyebrows may correctly prompt the examiner. The limbs may offer clues—broad or bifid halluces in **oro-facio-digital syndromes**, clinically confirmed by looking for multiple oral frenula, or ectrodactyly in **ectrodactyly-ectodermal dysplasia** syndrome. Sparse eyebrows and eyelashes and dry skin should result in evaluation of the parents for possible **Rapp-Hodgkin syndrome**, an autosomal dominant disorder, in which wiry hair, absence of secondary sexual hair, and hypohidrosis are usual. In boys, clefting associated with hypospadias or an ectopic anus is likely to signify **Opitz G syndrome**, and the possibility of laryngeal cleft needs to be formally investigated.

Investigations to Consider Karyotype is indicated only if there are additional unexplained malformations. Specific FISH for 4p16 in Wolf-Hirschhorn and molecular cytogenetic analysis may be necessary to identify subtle 1p36 deletion. The underlying loci are known for ectrodactyly-ectodermal dysplasia, Rapp-Hodgkin, Opitz G, and Van der Woude syndromes; the same is true of several holoprosencephaly loci, but the diagnosis is essentially a clinical issue.

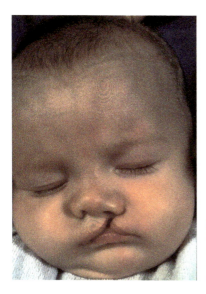

Figure 5.2A Unilateral cleft lip is seen in this patient. Note the secondary deformation of the nares consequent to the primary cleft malformation.

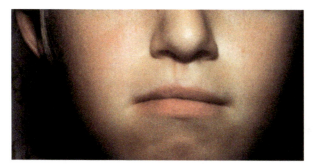

Figure 5.2B The vertical right-sided impression of a scar on this patient's philtrum is in fact a pseudocleft. He comes of a family with a strong history of autosomal dominant cleft lip and this clinical sign indicates that he carries the family mutation, though not affected as obviously as others in the pedigree.

5.3   Lip Pits

Recognizing the Sign   Three distinct forms are observed. Commisural pits, seen in the angles of the mouth on opening the oral cavity, are of no clinical significance. Upper lip pits generally occupy a midline situation and communicate with underlying glands but do not betoken a syndromic or dysmorphologic significance. Lower lip pits are generally seen as depressions, occasionally as minor elevations, on either side of the midline and also communicate with underlying glands. Most lower lip pits have a syndromic association.

Establishing a Differential Diagnosis   Lower lip pits are uncommon, the greatest hazard being that they are easily missed, and it is worth everting the lower lip to inspect the mucocutaneous junction for their presence. If observed, then three specific syndromes need to be considered in the course of examination. **Van der Woude syndrome** is an autosomal dominant condition, so a family history and examination of family members may further assist the diagnosis. Look for cleft palate, bifid or deviated uvula, and evidence of repaired cleft lip/palate in the family. Rare features described include Hirschsprung's disease and synechiae of the eyelids, but these are not typical. Cleft lip/palate and lip pits in the patient may signify **popliteal pterygium syndrome**, the clinical hallmark being popliteal webs, which limit extension of the knees. Since this syndrome is autosomal dominant, pertinent questioning with respect to the medical history of other family members will often generate additional diagnostic data. Good clinical clues to watch out for on examination are oligodactyly, syndactyly, hypoplastic nails, and genital malformations, especially micropenis. Finally, lip pits are an inconstant but valuable prompt to the sporadically occurring multiple congenital anomaly condition known as **Kabuki syndrome**. Characteristic facial features to look for in considering this diagnosis are arched eyebrows, often interrupted (in other words, a hairless region occurs as a gap in the eyebrow), and wide palpebral fissures, frequently with ectropion of the lower eyelid (Figure 3.14). Congenital heart defects are a common presentation in the newborn period and symptoms may be cardiac or feeding related, sustained feeding problems being a particular problem in these children. Variable immune dysfunction–related presentations in the first year or two of life are described, while presentation in the preschool child is generally related to delayed development. The history, facial features, and, if present, lip pits prompt the diagnosis. Confirmatory additional signs to be vigilant for during examination include fetal finger pads, blue sclera, and short stature. Obesity is a feature in adolescence.

Investigations to Consider   Analysis of the *IRF6* gene has established familial mutations in both Van der Woude and popliteal pterygium syndromes.

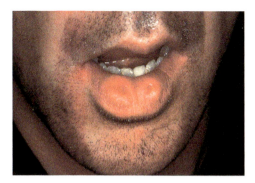

Figure 5.3A Slight swellings are shown on either side of the midline with the pits visible just behind the swellings. The patient has a diagnosis of Van der Woude syndrome.

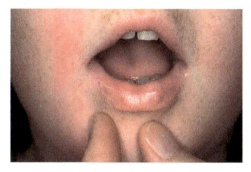

Figure 5.3B This photograph of a patient with Kabuki syndrome shows a pit as a slightly atrophic area on the patient's left.

5.4 Thick and Thin Upper Lips

Recognizing the Sign It is possible to formally measure the thickness of the lip. The *Handbook of Normal Physical Measurements* describes a technique measuring in the midline from the vermillion border to the aperture of the mouth and provides normal ranges. In practice, this is very rarely undertaken, but a subjective impression of the child's face may register the lip as being thicker or thinner than usual.

Establishing a Differential Diagnosis Unusual degrees of lip thickness can be familial and nonpathologic, so clinical signs relying on this observation are supportive of a diagnosis only in the presence of other concerns. Unusually thin lips noted in an older child under assessment for mild developmental delay or jitteriness in the newborn period may remind the examiner to consider **fetal alcohol syndrome** and other features of that ill-defined entity should be sought, such as microcephaly, unusual palmar creases, and a smooth philtrum. In assessing an older child presenting with short stature and mild developmental concerns, a thin upper lip may be the clue to a diagnosis of **Floating-Harbor syndrome**. Additional support for that conclusion would come from observing deep-set eyes and a nasal columella extending below the ala nasi and confirming from the history that the birth weight was low. When assessing a developmentally delayed child in whom there is a thick lip, be mindful in boys of the X-linked conditions **Coffin-Lowry syndrome** and **α-thalassemia mental retardation X syndrome** (ATRX). An especially valuable clinical sign in Coffin-Lowry patients are the fingers, which are puffy and tapering, sometimes described as "sausage shaped." Obviously a family history may offer consolidation, but examination of the mother can also be helpful—particularly the hands of carriers of Coffin-Lowry syndrome. Fullness of the lip is a helpful clinical feature of **Williams syndrome**, especially in the slightly older child, so it is worth checking the iris for a stellate pattern and the history for hypercalcemia or heart disease. Lip prominence in a newborn with unexplained growth retardation should cause the diagnosis of **leprechaunism** to be considered and provoke examination for the other clinical signs—acanthosis nigricans, breast enlargement, prominent ears, and genital enlargement.

Investigations to Consider Significant bone age delay is characteristic in Floating-Harbor syndrome. HbH inclusion bodies on brilliant cresyl blue staining are seen in about 90% of ATRX cases, though mutation analysis may sometimes be necessary to secure a diagnosis. Coffin-Lowry cases have mutations of the *RSK2* locus on Xp. Williams syndrome is confirmed by FISH for *ELN* deletion on 7q. Leprechaunism is confirmed by insulin receptor gene mutations, *INSR* on 19p.

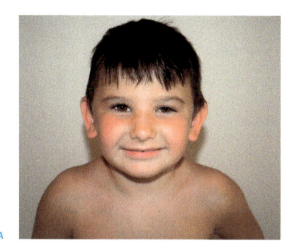

A

B

Figure 5.4A and B Thin upper lip (**A**) and brachyclinodactyly (**B**) are shown in this 5-year-old boy with Floating-Harbor syndrome, referred for developmental concerns and short stature. See Figures 9.9 for Coffin-Lowry syndrome and Figure 1.6C for ATRX syndrome.

5.5 Lip and Oral Mucosa Pigmentation

Recognizing the Sign Spotty pigmentation of the lips and oral mucosa is an uncommon finding with very specific clinical connotations. The sign is readily recognizable as brownish macules, of variable diameter, most noticeable on the lips but sometimes also present on the hard palate, gums, oral mucosa, and perioral and periorbital regions. Very infrequent at birth or in the newborn period, these usually develop in later childhood.

Establishing a Differential Diagnosis The family history may betray clues—**neurofibromatosis type 1** is a good example, where the emergence of clinical features in a child takes place over a period of time but the diagnosis can generally be suspected and complications sought early by reference to family history. Assess carefully for optic glioma in the young child and for scoliosis in the older age group. Blood pressure monitoring is important in all age groups, there being an association with both pheochromocytoma and renal artery stenosis. The classical association of lip pigmentation is **Peutz-Jeghers syndrome** (P-JS), in which hamartomatous polyposis and malignant propensity of the small bowel is increased, as are malignancies of the breasts and reproductive organs. Episodic colicky abdominal pain in adolescence usually signals intussusception of small bowel polyps. Macules may also be found on the palms, soles, volar aspects of the fingers, and genitalia. **Laugier-Hunziker syndrome** (L-HS) is a very rare, sporadic condition clinically indistinguishable from P-JS in lip and oral pigmentation, but without associated gastrointestinal complication. Whereas the onset of the pigmentation in P-JS is usually complete by puberty, the onset of pigmentation in L-HS is usually in adult life. In **Carney complex**, the lip and mucosal pigmentation is spotty, but usually has a more extensive distribution around the face. This autosomal dominant diagnosis is important because of the association with atrial myxoma. Conjunctival pigmentation and eyelid myxomas are occasional features. Finally, consider **LEOPARD syndrome** (*l*entigines, *e*chocardiographic abnormalities, *o*cular hypertelorism, *p*ulmonary stenosis, *a*bnormal genitalia, *r*etardation of growth, and *d*eafness). Assess for hypospadias, cardiac murmurs, and multiple lentigines of the face, neck, and trunk, and assess parents for evidence of this autosomal dominant condition.

Investigations to Consider Almost all cases can be resolved at a clinical level. Echocardiography is important for LEOPARD and Carney complex, to specifically assess for atrial myxomata in the latter disorder, which may be recurrent. Mutation analysis is available for all conditions in the event of clinical uncertainty.

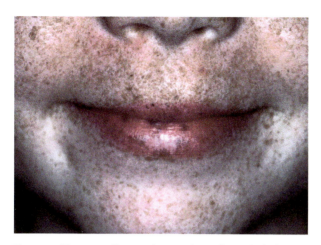

Figure 5.5 Numerous discrete pigmented macules, typical of Peutz-Jeghers syndrome, are demonstrated.

5.6 Macroglossia

Recognizing the Sign The tongue is usually contained fully within the oral cavity, and any protrusion of the tongue begs examination. True macroglossia signifies a large tongue, while relative macroglossia signifies a small oral cavity, the tongue protrusion being a secondary effect.

Establishing a Differential Diagnosis Establish whether there is micrognathia, a clue that the macroglossia is secondary. In the neonate, specifically examine for clinical signs of **Down syndrome**—especially useful are hypotonia, poor Moro reflex, excess nuchal skin, and simian hand creases. In the older child whose chromosomes are normal but whose development is inexplicably delayed, relative macroglossia and a flat or dished appearance to the midface can be the clues to **chromosome 9q34 deletion** syndrome. The clinical impression of the 9q34-deleted patient among colleagues and family is often of a patient who looks like he or she has Down syndrome but who has "normal" chromosomes. True macroglossia in the neonate is suggestive of **Beckwith-Wiedemann syndrome** (BWS). Corroborative signs to look out for are nevus flammeus, visceromegaly, ear creases on the lobe or pit-like depressions on the helical rim, a history of hypoglycemia, and a history of assisted conception, which is associated with increased prevalence of BWS. There is clinical overlap between BWS and **Simpson-Golabi-Behmel syndrome**, an X-linked mental retardation syndrome comprising large birth weight and macroglossia, often with a deep midline groove on the tongue, the groove perhaps extending to the lower lip. Particularly valuable clinical signs that suggest this diagnosis are accessory nipples and nail hypoplasia, most notably of the index finger. Asymmetry of a congenitally enlarged tongue probably signifies an underlying **hemihypertrophy** as the cause, and careful examination of the limbs may show evidence for this. Macroglossia in a neonate whose clinical presentation is of unexplained weakness and/or poor feeding is typical of **Pompe's disease**, a glycogen storage disorder. Tongue fasciculation and joint contractures are corroborative signs to assess. An impression of macroglossia combined with emerging developmental concerns in the first couple of months of life should prompt investigation of **mucopolysaccharidosis** (MCP), even before other clinical signs such as joint stiffness and corneal clouding appear.

Investigations to Consider Karyotype is indicated for suspected Down syndrome, but specific molecular cytogenetic assay is required to identify 9q34 deletion. BWS remains in essence a clinical diagnosis, molecular analysis for 11p imprinting center defects being demonstrable in about 50% of cases. Simpson-Golabi-Behmel syndrome may be confirmed by mutation analysis of the *GPC3* gene on Xq21. An electrocardiogram is valuable in Pompe's disease, showing giant QRS complexes, and an echocardiograph shows ventricular enlargement. Glycosaminoglycan excretion in urine is the screening test for MCP.

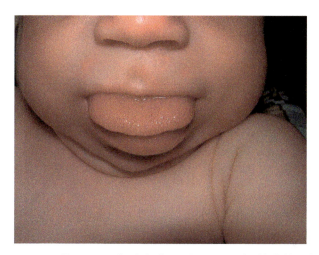

Figure 5.6 True macroglossia is shown in a 3-month-old child with Beckwith-Wiedemann syndrome, conceived by assisted reproduction.

5.7 Accessory Oral Frenula

Recognizing the Sign The frenula are the normal folds of mucosal membrane extending between the alveolar ridge and the inside of the upper lip and the counterparts inside the lower lip and beneath the tongue. Any additional such mucosal folds are termed accessory frenula or aberrant frenula.

Establishing a Differential Diagnosis Accessory frenula are important clues to syndrome diagnosis but are not the subject of scrutiny in most general clinical examinations undertaken and, for this reason, are often found in children whose more clinically obvious signs have been noted earlier. In a newborn with postaxial polydactyly of the hands, the identification of accessory oral frenula is very suggestive of the autosomal recessive condition **Ellis-van Creveld syndrome**. Look for corroborative signs, especially small, deep-set, hypoplastic fingernails and a murmur consistent with an atrial septal defect, present in about 50% of cases. Natal teeth are another good clue to this diagnosis on intraoral examination, though not invariable. The presence of cleft lip or palate should prompt a search for lip pits and accessory frenula, which are common in **popliteal pterygium syndrome**. The pterygia result in a popliteal web and there is associated abnormality of the toenail of the hallux, a pyramidal skinfold extending from the base to the tip of the toenails. The clinical value of limb assessment also applies to **hypoglossia-hypodactyly syndrome**, in which a small tongue is seen, often with accessory oral frenula, perhaps extending between the palate and the floor of the mouth. There is associated micrognathia, and cranial nerve defects, especially of the sixth and seventh nerves, are often demonstrable clinically. Syndactyly, adactyly, and variable microdactyly should be sought. In **oro-facio-digital (OFD) syndromes**, of which there are a bewildering variety of clinically and genetically distinct forms, oral frenula associated with preaxial or postaxial polydactyly signal the diagnosis. Though not invariable, mental retardation in associated with several forms of OFD syndromes, as are central nervous system malformations.

Investigations to Consider Karyotype is justified if accessory frenula are identified as part of a child with multiple congenital anomalies for whom no unifying syndromic diagnosis is apparent. Neuroimaging of the brain is important in refining the diagnosis of which form of OFD syndrome a child may have, the inheritance differing among the several discrete forms. Mutation analysis for Ellis-van Creveld and popliteal pterygium syndromes is not necessary to the diagnosis of these clinically recognizable disorders.

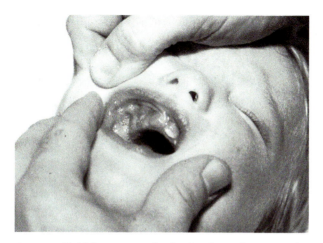

Figure 5.7 Multiple accessory alveolar frenula are demonstrated in this patient with a diagnosis of orofaciodigital syndrome, type II. Note the associated gum hypertrophy, which was secondary to phenytoin medication for epilepsy. (Reproduced with permission from Reardon et al., *J Med Genet* 1989;26:659–663.)

5.8 Isolated Cleft Palate

Recognizing the Sign Cleft of the soft and/or hard palate is easily seen and should be sought in all infants. Less easily identified are more subtle forms, specifically submucous clefting of the soft palate, wherein the oral mucosa shows no defect but a notch is palpable at the posterior margin of the hard palate. The uvula should always be inspected and, if bifid, a submucous cleft should be suspected. The associated velopharyngeal incompetence may be suspected in a baby where a history of milk leaking down the nares during feeding is elicited. Recourse to examination by an expert may be required to confirm.

Establishing a Differential Diagnosis Fifty percent of cases of isolated cleft palate have associated congenital malformations and 20% have an identifiable monogenic cause, while 1% of cases have a chromosomal abnormality. **Trisomy 13** represents the most recognizable karyotypic abnormality, but very many others are described. However, most cleft palate cases are isolated events often associated with micrognathia, resulting in Pierre-Robin sequence. In seeking monogenic causes, the family history may indicate several affected males in a kindred, suggesting the nonsyndromic condition of **X-linked cleft palate**. Ankyloglossia, where the tongue is anchored to the floor of the mouth, is a feature in some individuals affected with this disorder, while female heterozygotes may show bifid uvula and submucous clefting. Lip pits or cleft lip in the family should suggest **Van der Woude syndrome** (section 5.3). A cardiac murmur clinically in a child with cleft palate or a history suggestive of velopharyngeal incompetence should prompt assessment for **velo-cardio-facial** (VCF) syndrome. Look for the prominent nose, the nasal tip being somewhat square, and seek a corroborative history of hypocalcemia or recurrent infections. VCF syndrome is remarkably variable, and a low threshold for investigation is appropriate. Hypospadias associated with cleft palate, especially if there is a family history of same, is likely to signify the X-linked condition of **Opitz G syndrome**. Female heterozygotes may show mild degrees of hypertelorism. Severe short stature present at birth with nasal flattening and associated cleft palate points toward a skeletal dysplasia as the underlying cause, the exact diagnosis possibly being **Kniest syndrome**. Joint laxity in association with cleft palate may be symptomatic of **Stickler syndrome**, especially if there is evidence of myopia and flattening of the nasal bridge.

Investigations to Consider Karyotype is almost always normal, but FISH of 22q11 is important for diagnosis of VCF cases. Skeletal radiology in association with clinical findings is the basis of Kniest and Stickler diagnoses.

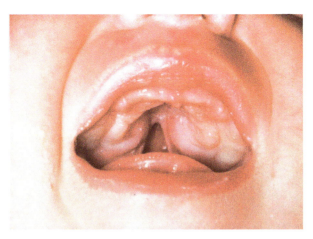

Figure 5.8A The typical V-shaped defect in the soft palate is demonstrated in this child who had no other malformations and for whom a diagnosis of nonsyndromic cleft palate was reached.

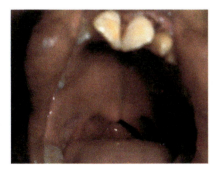

Figure 5.8B Absent uvula with associated mid-line translucency, betraying absence of muscle fusion, is shown. These features are entirely consistent with a diagnosis of subclinical cleft palate. (Courtesy of Mr. David Orr.)

5.9 Persistent Drooling

Recognizing the Sign This hardly requires any clinical expertise, but a good history can inform the examination and investigation. The neonatal feeding history will often be of a poor feeding pattern, perhaps requiring nasogastric supplementation. Establish whether there was macroglossia at birth, cleft palate, or micrognathia. Was there any suggestion of velopharyngeal incompetence on feeding, often represented by nasal regurgitation of milk during feeding? Gauge the progress of the child with respect to perceptive and expressive speech.

Establishing a Differential Diagnosis Observe the face for evidence of a generalized **myopathy** and then assess the patient's muscle bulk generally. Specifically, look at the tongue. Establish whether it looks large and symmetric, perhaps with a deep central groove, which might cause you to consider **Simpson-Golabi-Behmel (SGB) syndrome**, especially if there was a high birth weight, a history of X-linked mental retardation, and/or cardiac malformations. Evaluate the heart clinically—a murmur will add weight to your diagnostic concern. Cardiac concerns, a history of nasal regurgitation of milk on feeding, and speech delay may equate with **velo-cardio-facial** (VCF) syndrome. Does the tongue look asymmetric, in which case careful evaluation of the face and limbs for asymmetry is warranted? Does the tongue move normally and specifically assess whether the child protrudes the tongue from the oral cavity? Failure to protrude the tongue with a history of poor feeding and delayed expressive speech is typical of **Worster-Drought syndrome**. In this condition, examine the lower cranial nerves—often there are signs of pseudobulbar palsy. There may be a striking discrepancy between the general development of the child, which can be within normal parameters, and the expressive speech, which is greatly delayed. A history of polyhydramnios, an open-mouth appearance, and generalized muscle weakness are the classic hallmarks of **congenital myotonic dystrophy**. Careful evaluation of the family history may establish cases of symptomatic cataract before the age of 40 years, and maternal examination in this condition will establish corroborative signs, such as myotonia of the thenar eminence on percussion. Transmission of the congenital form is virtually exclusively maternal. Sixth or seventh cranial nerve palsy strongly suggests **Moebius syndrome** as the underlying diagnosis, in which case limb asymmetry, syndactyly, and brachydactyly should be sought and the pectoral wall muscles be evaluated, since absence is quite common in this condition.

Investigations to Consider *GPC3* gene mutations underlie SGB syndrome, but clinical diagnosis is usually possible. FISH of 22q11 is indicated to establish VCF syndrome. Myotonic dystrophy is demonstrable as a triplet repeat expansion in the *MD* gene on chromosome 19. Magnetic resonance imaging scan in Worster-Drought cases frequently establishes perisylvian polymicrogyria.

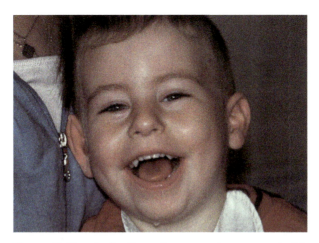

Figure 5.9A Note the drooling and open-mouth appearance in this 3-year-old boy referred for "unexplained mental retardation." The motor milestones were almost within normal parameters, but he had persistent drooling and could not protrude his tongue. A clinical diagnosis of Worster-Drought syndrome was made.

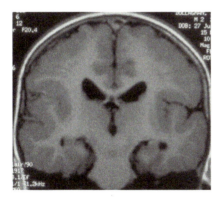

Figure 5.9B Magnetic resonance imaging scan of the same patient confirms perisylvian polymicrogyria.

5.10　Gum Hyperplasia

Recognizing the Sign　In the child whose teeth have erupted, gum hypertrophy is readily apparent, the teeth being engulfed by the gingiva, which may themselves have a nodular appearance. In the neonate, this clinical sign is much more subjective. Repeated observation of the normal during routine examination will develop the necessary recognition skills to identify the abnormal.

Establishing a Differential Diagnosis　The most commonly recognized cause of gingival hyperplasia is drug related and a history of medications taken may readily explain the clinical sign. Specifically, **phenytoin** and **cyclosporin** are medications that are commonly associated with this clinical side effect. The observation of gum hyperplasia in the neonatal stage suggests a few specific diagnoses—Robinow syndrome, I-cell disease, and **leprechaunism**. In the latter, breast enlargement, genital hypertrophy, and acanthosis nigricans strongly support this possible diagnosis, especially if there is a history of intrauterine growth retardation and a general appearance of lipodystrophy—very little subcutaneous fat. Clinical features that ought to be sought in **Robinow syndrome** include cleft lip, anteverted nares, and hypertelorism. The genitalia may not be notably abnormal in the female, but a normally formed small penis is usual in affected males. It is worth noting the hands and feet—if there is not clinical evidence of a bifid thumb or hallux, a broad digit may be the prompt that radiologic investigation might establish evidence of incomplete reduplication. **I-cell disease** follows a typical storage disease pattern, with concerns that development is not proceeding normally often prompted by initial feeding difficulties, progressive limitation of joint movement, and corneal clouding. The author has seen the diagnosis made prior to the emergence of any of these landmarks by preemptive investigation following the recognition of gum hyperplasia in the neonate. There is clinical overlap between I-cell disease and a rare autosomal recessive disorder, **infantile systemic hyalinosis**, in which failure to thrive neonatally, gingival hyperplasia, and crying due to pain on joint movement, with the early emergence of flexion contractures, represent a fairly typical pattern. Facial papules, perioral pigmentation, and fleshy nodules at the anal margin allow this condition to be confidently recognized. Hyperpigmented swellings over the metacarpophalangeal joints emerge with time.

Investigations to Consider　Hemivertebrae or bifid terminal phalanges of the thumb/hallux radiologically support the clinical diagnosis of Robinow syndrome. Insulin receptor gene mutations confirm leprechaunism, if the clinical diagnosis is not secure. While urinary oligosaccharides, vacuolated lymphocytes, and/or disordered lysosomal enzymes may be observed in I-cell disease, fibroblast culture is required for demonstration of the characteristic "inclusion bodies."

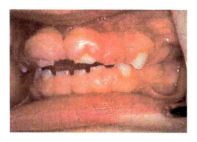

Figure 5.10A Gum hypertrophy in a 6-year-old child treated with cyclosporin. (Courtesy of Mr. Paddy Fleming.)

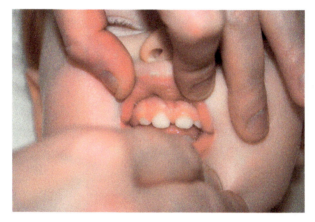

Figure 5.10B Gum hypertrophy in a 14-month-old child with I-cell disease.

Chapter 6   The Neck

6.1 Neck Webbing

Recognizing the Sign Neck webbing refers to redundant skin at the back and sides of the neck and is thought to arise from resolved nuchal edema in utero. In contrast to a short neck, it is possible to palpate the folds of excess skin between the fingers. The posterior hairline is often extended downward in association with the webs of excess skin. Distinction needs to be drawn between excess nuchal skin and specific webs of tissue (pterygia) in the neck region, which frequently accompany limitation of extension in multiple joints as part of a wider multiple pterygium syndrome, all of them rare.

Establishing a Differential Diagnosis Observe the parents and ask if either of them have needed cardiac examination/intervention. **Noonan syndrome** frequently presents with nuchal edema, indeed even generalized hydrops on occasion, and much negative investigation may be spared by such parental evaluation. Short stature, ptosis, and posteriorly rotated ears are all good clinical signs to watch out for in considering this diagnosis, as well as a cardiac examination for congenital heart disease, particularly pulmonary stenosis. A history of abnormal bleeding after minor procedures is consistent with Noonan syndrome. In the older child, multiple café-au-lait patches with facial and other features of Noonan syndrome signify the subtype known as **Noonan-neurofibromatosis type 1** (NF1). These children essentially have NF1 and need appropriate management measures for that condition. Clinical signs of coarctation of the aorta in a baby with excess nuchal skin should cause a likely diagnosis of **Turner syndrome** to be considered. The classic clinical signs of cubitus valgus, short stature, and wide-spaced nipples may not be apparent until much later, but puffy feet are a good clue in the neonate. Excess nuchal skin may occur as part of a generalized cutis laxa presentation. Early feeding difficulties may presage the later emergence of coarse facial features, developmental delay, and a diagnosis of **Costello syndrome**. Likewise, a generalized cutis laxa presentation, but with normal development, can signal a connective tissue disorder, most likely one of the forms of **Ehlers-Danlos syndrome** (EDS). Assessment should establish the degree of skin elasticity as well as any scarring, striae, easy bruising, and a family history of the same.

Investigations to Consider An echocardiogram is mandatory if a diagnosis of Noonan or Turner syndrome is being considered. Costello syndrome is open to molecular investigation of the *KRAS* gene but this is rarely necessary in experienced clinical hands. Before reaching a diagnosis of EDS, it is worth assaying tenascin X, easily done on serum, deficiency of which produces a condition that overlaps with EDS, especially types II and III.

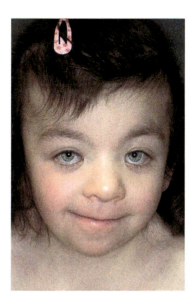

Figure 6.1 Excess nuchal skin is demonstrated in this girl with Noonan syndrome, whose neonatal presentation was of generalized hydrops.

6.2 Short Neck

Recognizing the Sign The underlying problem in this clinical situation is likely malformation or malsegmentation of the cervical vertebrae. Consequently, the head appears to sit directly on the shoulders. Unsurprisingly, the posterior hairline is usually low and the mobility of the neck reduced in all directions. Neck webbing may be observed as an associated secondary phenomenon.

Establishing a Differential Diagnosis Empirically, the most likely diagnosis is that of **Klippel-Feil syndrome**. In this condition, there will be an underlying radiologic fusion of vertebrae, which may extend beyond the cervical region in severe cases. Clinical examination should assess for evidence of a sixth cranial nerve palsy (Duane phenomenon) and deafness, both associated with Klippel-Feil malformation, the combination of all three being known as Wildervanck syndrome. Curiously, the condition is almost exclusive to females. Associated malformations of the renal and internal genital tracts are common, specifically vaginal atresia, absent uterus, renal agenesis, hypoplasia, and ureteric reduplication. Mirror movements are a well-described clinical phenomenon and should be sought. Epibulbar dermoids should be noted, and their observation supports the likely diagnosis. Congenital upward displacement of the scapula, known as Sprengel shoulder, may be unilaterally or bilaterally present. The observation of a short neck and/or Sprengel shoulder in a male should be followed by palpation of the vas deferens, **congenital bilateral absence of the vasa** being a frequent phenomenon in boys with renal anomalies and cervical malsegmentation. The association of limb abnormalities, especially thenar eminence hypoplasia or thumb reduplication, is more reminiscent of **MURCS association** (Müllerian, renal, cervical spine), in which the vertebral fusion is associated with renal and uterine dysplasia, generally with absence of the uterus. In the event of a short neck being observed in a child of normal developmental progress but concerns of short stature, it is useful to be aware that **Morquio syndrome** (mucopolysaccharidosis [MPS] type IV) may so present, the limitation of joint movement characteristic of other types of MPS not being so reliable in this form of storage disease. Corneal clouding and opacities should be sought, but are not invariable.

Investigations to Consider Neck radiology and renal and pelvic ultrasound are essential to fully evaluate Klippel-Feil and associated malformations, and likewise to differentiate MURCS syndrome. Audiologic evaluation should be considered. Keratan sulphate urinary excretion is usually increased in MPS type IV. Skeletal radiology will generally show dysostosis multiplex, and odontoid hypoplasia is a particular feature. Enzymatic confirmation is available by leucocyte study.

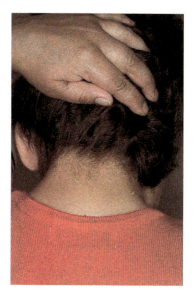

Figure 6.2 Short neck and low posterior hairline are shown in a female patient who presented at age 14 years, with short stature and menstruation not having commenced. The uterus was absent. There was unilateral renal agenesis and cervical vertebrae C3–5 were fused. The diagnosis was MURCS association.

6.3 Goiter

Recognizing the Sign Goiter simply signifies enlargement of the thyroid. Generally in children this is of uniform, as opposed to nodular or localized, character, as can apply in adults. The bilobar shape of the thyroid, straddling the midline, is readily apparent.

Establishing a Differential Diagnosis Neonatal goiter is uncommon and should rightly raise concerns for a biochemical abnormality in thyroxine synthesis. However, do be aware that **maternal ingestion of carbimazole** can result in congenital goiter. In the event of a maternal history of carbimazole ingestion, it is worth looking specifically for choanal atresia, or severe narrowing of the nasal passages, as well as nipple hypoplasia or absence in the baby, both features well described in carbimazole embryopathy. Likewise, localized scalp defects have been described in several cases of this teratogenesis syndrome. In considering possible **metabolic causes**, it is worth recording that most causes of neonatal hypothyroidism are associated with aplasia or aberrant development of the gland and will not be associated with goiter. However, congenital or emerging neonatal goiter does require full pituitary evaluation, lest a treatable form of mental retardation be missed. Oral thyroxine is effective in such cases. The most common association of childhood goiter is with **Pendred syndrome**, in which deafness is the key feature. Generally the deafness predates the onset of goiter by a decade or more. The deafness has particular characteristics that allow the diagnosis to be suspected clinically. The hearing threshold fluctuates and parents will be aware of day-to-day variation in the child's hearing; it is sensitive to atmospheric pressure variation, so it can deteriorate after airline travel, diving, etc., and it is often associated with variable vestibular symptoms. Acute, irreversible loss of hearing following head injury is well described. If the deafness has been appropriately evaluated by computed tomography (CT) scan of the petrous temporal bones, the diagnosis will be made well before the thyroid enlargement emerges—typically in the second decade of life. Congenital and early-onset goiter is very uncommon in Pendred syndrome.

Investigations to Consider Thyroid-stimulating hormone (TSH) evaluation, thyroid-releasing hormone (TRH) stimulation, and magnetic resonance imaging (MRI) evaluation of the anterior pituitary are urgent considerations in congenital goiter. In the deaf child, dilatation of the vestibular aqueducts, on CT scan of the petrous temporal bones, will disclose the very likely diagnosis of Pendred syndrome. The only other documented cause of dilated vestibular aqueduct as an isolated finding is distal renal tubular acidosis with deafness. Less commonly, a Mondini malformation of the cochlea is identified in Pendred syndrome patients. Mutation analysis of the *SLC26A4* gene discloses multiple mutations in both goiter-associated and non–goiter-associated Pendred syndrome.

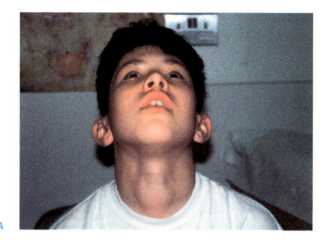

A

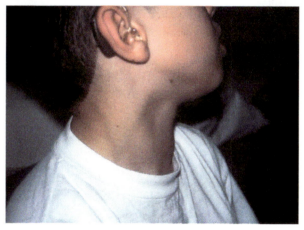

B

Figure 6.3A and B The diffuse swelling in the neck in this deaf patient betrays the underlying diagnosis of Pendred syndrome. The deafness was recognized early, the goiter becoming apparent at age 12 years.

6.4 Neck Sinuses/Fistulae/Pits

Recognizing the Sign A clinical distinction between a branchial sinus and a fistula cannot be drawn without surgical exploration. By definition, a fistula has an external opening onto the cutaneous surface and extends inward, opening into the pharynx. A sinus, by contrast, is blind ending internally but, like a fistula, creates a clinically identifiable pit on the skin. These external openings are generally seen along the anterior border of the sternocleido-mastoid muscle and are sometimes a focus for secretions and secondary infection. The only other likely cause of a neck sinus is a thyroglossal cyst, which, by contrast to branchial cysts/sinuses, is midline and may be found at any position between the sternal notch and the hyoid bone.

Establishing a Differential Diagnosis Thyroglossal cysts, though occasion-ally familial, do not betoken a syndromic association and should be viewed as isolated developmental malformations. Branchial pits need more careful di-agnostic evaluation. Most occur as sporadic isolated findings, either unilateral or bilateral, in otherwise normal individuals, without evidence of associated malformations. The specific diagnostic concern raised by the observation of a branchial sinus is whether the patient has **branchio-oto-renal (BOR) syn-drome**. Preauricular pits; external ear malformations, including microtia; and evidence of deafness should be assessed. Most affected individuals have hearing loss, with mixed type being most likely. The external auditory canal is often narrow; indeed, cholesteatoma is occasionally described. A history of urinary tract infection will suggest renal involvement and needs to be specifi-cally investigated, irrespective of symptoms, if this diagnosis is under consid-eration. Renal agenesis or hypoplasia, cystic renal changes, and vesicoureteric reflux are all described, though actual renal failure is rare. The identification of a sixth nerve palsy is specific to deletions involving the BOR locus on chro-mosome 8. Neck sinuses overlying a hemangiomatous region of tissue, often along the line of the sternocleidomastoid muscle but also occurring behind the ear, are typical of **branchio-oculo-facial (BOF) syndrome**. The philtrum is narrow but shows thick vertical ridges, producing a pseudocleft appearance. Ocular involvement is usual and can embrace coloboma, lacrimal gland ob-struction, and hypertelorism separately or in combination.

Investigations to Consider Biochemical parameters of renal function should be undertaken in both BOR and BOF syndromes as well as ultrasound eval-uation of the kidneys and renal tract. CT scan of the petrous temporal bone in BOR syndrome shows dilated vestibular aqueduct in association with mid-dle ear malformations, including ossicular anomalies. Mutations of the *EYA1* locus on chromosome 8 are demonstrable but rarely necessary to secure the diagnosis. Patients with Duane syndrome (sixth nerve palsy) need detailed evaluation molecularly for chromosome 8q deletion.

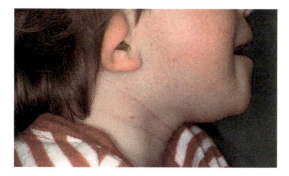

Figure 6.4A A typical branchial sinus is shown from a patient with BOR syndrome. Note also the lop ear.

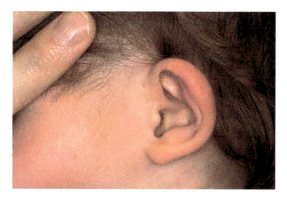

Figure 6.4B The contralateral ear in the same patient demonstrates the characteristic site of preauricular pit in BOR syndrome.

6.5 Occipital Horns

Recognizing the Sign The term reflects occipital exostoses due to calcification of the trapezius and sternocleidomastoid muscles at their attachment to the occipital bone. This is not a sign identifiable in infancy or early childhood, taking some years to become apparent, but when they occur, occipital horns are clinically apparent on palpation before the age of 10 years and, radiologically, are identifiable earlier.

Establishing a Differential Diagnosis The phenomenon of a clinical sign being "pathognomonic" or signaling one condition exclusively is quite rare in syndromology, but does apply to occipital horns. This clinical sign is exclusive to the condition known as **occipital horn syndrome**, which is synonymous with Ehlers-Danlos syndrome type IX. Slight ptosis, generalized skin laxity, easy bruising, and hyperextensible joints, perhaps occasioning delay in walking, will allow early classification of the patient as likely to represent some form of Ehlers-Danlos syndrome. Being X-linked, all affected individuals are male. The family history may offer a clue to the true diagnosis before the occipital horns become apparent. Most affected individuals are mildly mentally retarded, and occasional instances associated with epilepsy are recorded. Other useful clinical signs that betray the true diagnosis to the alert clinician are the long neck and trunk, pes planus, and genu valgum. An early history of inguinal hernia is common, and bladder diverticula resulting in intermittent outlet obstruction or recurrent infections are well described. Diarrhea of unknown origin is also recognized.

Investigations to Consider Hair microscopy may reveal pili torti, in which the shaft of the hair is rotated 180 degrees along the longitudinal axis. Though neither consistent nor diagnostic, serum copper levels are usually reduced. Skeletal x-rays, in addition to the occipital horns, may show short, broad clavicles and carpal fusion. Fibroblast evaluation of copper metabolism typically shows an increased concentration of intracellular copper. The ultimate confirmation of this condition, which is difficult to diagnose prior to the identification of the pathognomonic clinical sign, is mutation demonstration in the *MKS* Menkes syndrome gene on Xq12. The disease is allelic with Menkes syndrome.

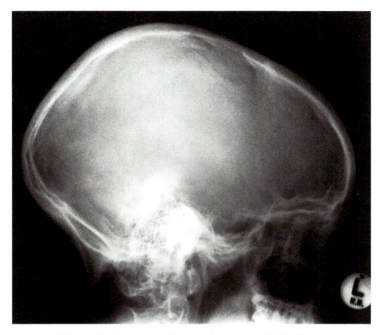

Figure 6.5 The occipital exostoses that give rise to the palpable "horns" are demonstrated.

Chapter 7   **The Chest**

7.1 Poland Anomaly

Recognizing the Sign The essential issue is absence or hypoplasia of the sternal head of the pectoralis major muscle. Hence, the recognition will be triggered by upper chest asymmetry and absence of the usual anterior axillary fold. If in doubt, get the patient to place the hand on the hip and contract the muscle, which facilitates easy palpation of the muscle bulk at the anterior axilla. Breast asymmetry is often an easy clue to the muscle hypoplasia. Examine the hands for the brachydactyly and/or syndactyly, which frequently accompanies the chest malformation. Typically there is hypoplasia of the middle phalanges, often with fusion of the terminal phalanges and skin syndactyly. Fifth finger clinodactyly is usual but the thumb is generally fairly normal. Muscle bulk in the arms/forearms may be asymmetric. These observations are almost always unilateral and on the same side as the chest muscle defect.

Establishing a Differential Diagnosis Assess the heart, as there is an association with dextrocardia. More important in terms of cardiac function, there is an association with subclavian artery stenosis and aberrant arterial supply, so assessment of the pulses in the neck and arms may be useful. Cardiac and upper limb involvement can overlap clinically with the spectrum of abnormalities comprising **Holt-Oram syndrome** (H-OS), an autosomal dominant disorder of variable cardiac malformation but most commonly causing atrial septal defects, which also involves pectoral muscles in a minority of cases. Accordingly, family history, parental history of congenital heart disease, and cardiac assessment can have a significant impact on the interpretation of what may initially appear to be a curiosity of isolated malformation. However, most cases of pure Poland anomaly are sporadic events. Holt-Oram syndrome aside, the other main diagnostic consideration is the condition known as **Poland-Moebius syndrome**, in which disorder the typical chest and hand malformations of Poland anomaly are associated with congenital bilateral sixth and seventh cranial nerve palsy. Careful evaluation of the lower cranial nerves is indicated, as the neural deficit can often involve the bulbar region. Mental retardation is relatively uncommon (5%–10%).

Investigations to Consider The presence of Poland signs in cases of Moebius is important because it effectively reassures the clinician that the Moebius signs are not related to a primary muscle pathology. Moebius syndrome without Poland signs requires more extensive muscle investigation, including electrical evaluation. Echocardiography and, in occasional cases, angiocardiography comprise the mainstay of investigation in Poland anomaly. Genetic investigations are not indicated.

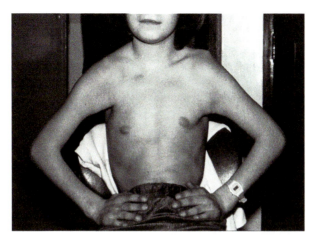

Figure 7.1A The right-sided deficiency of the pectoralis major muscle is reflected in the breast asymmetry, the sloping shoulder, and the line of the anterior axillary wall. This patient also had ipsilateral 3/4 syndactyly. (Reproduced with permission from Reardon et al. *Clin Genet* 1990;38:233–236.)

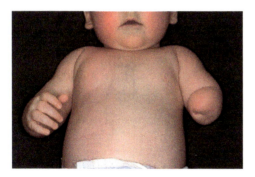

Figure 7.1B This photograph shows a left-sided limb hemimelia, a rare complication of Poland anomaly. More important diagnostically is the observation that the inframammary crease is clearly seen on the right side and is absent on the left side and there is asymmetry of the anterior axillary skin creases, betraying the left-sided pectoral muscle deficiency.

7.2 Accessory Nipples

Recognizing the Sign Most commonly sited inferior and medial to the normal nipple, supernumerary nipples may be identified by their presentation as small pigmented marks or as dimples. They may be confused with birthmarks, moles, or nevi. Some 60% show a unilateral single additional nipple, 30% demonstrate bilaterality, and the remainder show three or more additional nipples. Mostly these arise as an isolated clinical finding and are devoid of further significance.

Establishing a Differential Diagnosis It is worth being aware that the feature can be inherited as an uncomplicated autosomal dominant trait and also that a specific association with renal tract anomalies is described, embracing hypoplastic kidneys, ectopic kidneys, collection system reduplication, etc. Since the feature is an occasional finding in **fetal valproate** exposure in utero, a drug history in pregnancy may offer an explanation. Specific genetic syndromes in which accessory nipples are identified such as **Rubinstein-Taybi syndrome** and **Miller syndrome** will be more easily identified by their signature clinical features of broad thumb and prominent beaked nose in the former and malar hypoplasia with postaxial limb defects in the latter. However, there are several syndromes associated with accessory nipples in which this clinical finding may serve as the clue to the underlying diagnosis. Primary among these is **Pallister-Killian syndrome** (tetrasomy 12p), a condition that should be sought in situations of emerging developmental concerns, often associated with seizures and an early history of hypotonia. Macroglossia and poor hair growth in the temporal regions are valuable clinical signs. Examination under ultraviolet light may show areas of patchy hypopigmentation, signifying mosaicism. **Simpson-Golabi-Behmel syndrome** is an X-linked overgrowth condition often associated with additional nipples. A family history, especially of high birth weight, postaxial polydactyly, and mild developmental delay, will all sharpen the likelihood of this underlying disorder in a child with supernumerary nipples. Hypertelorism; a deep midline groove on the tongue, lower lip; and chin; and hypoplasia of the index fingernail are all diagnostically supportive clinical signs to watch out for. Macrocephaly, a family history of the same, lipomata, and mental retardation in association with accessory nipples should lead to investigation for **Bannayan-Zonana syndrome**.

Investigations to Consider Chromosomal analysis on skin fibroblasts is usually necessary to demonstrate the tetrasomy of chromosome 12p in Pallister-Killian syndrome, though repeat biopsies may be required. Melanocyte culture is reputed to be more reliable, though very infrequently available. Mutation analysis of the *GPC3* gene is available for Simpson-Golabi-Behmel confirmation and of *PTen* for Bannayan-Zonana and overlapping phenotypes.

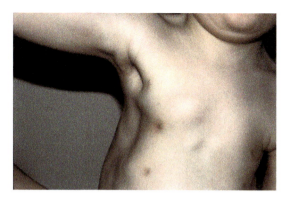

Figure 7.2 This patient shows accessory nipples bilaterally, in the midline, but also has accessory nipples at the anterior axillary wall, which is demonstrated on the right side. Though present on the left side also, the accessory nipple is obscured by the skin creases of the axillary wall.

7.3 Athelia/Hypothelia (Absent or Hypoplastic Nipples)

Recognizing the Sign Absence of the nipple is easily recognized in infancy and is generally associated with amastia of the breast tissue, which will not become apparent in the female until puberty. Hypoplasia of the nipple is more difficult to recognize, but should be considered if there is little pigment around the nipple and if the areola, which should underlie and surround the nipple, is absent. The remarks appertaining to Poland anomaly (section 7.1) apply. Assess the chest wall musculature, facial movement, and ipsilateral upper limb. In the event of these being normal, consider the following possibilities.

Establishing a Differential Diagnosis Family history can be diagnostically significant because both autosomal dominant and recessive forms of athelia are described, as isolated findings. Likewise, a detailed history of drug ingestion can solve the diagnostic mystery, with **carbimazole**, widely used for treatment of thyrotoxicosis in pregnancy, being associated with absent or hypoplastic nipples, often in association with choanal atresia. Scalp defects and imperforate anus are also described in this syndrome of teratogenesis. **Chromosomal aneuploidies** can result in this clinical sign, but almost always in the context of a more significant multiorgan malformation complex. Specifically, Edwards syndrome (trisomy 18) is often associated with nipple hypoplasia. Likewise, though a common feature of de Lange syndrome, the diagnosis will be signaled by the characteristic facial and limb findings outlined elsewhere. Small, invariably inverted nipples are important diagnostic clues to the **carbohydrate-deficient glycoprotein (CDG) syndromes**. Other clinical clues include unusual fat pad distribution over the buttocks and areas of lipoatrophy. With time, developmental delay is noted and, later, cerebellar ataxia can emerge as an important clue to etiology. Limb defects, typically deficient digits on the ulnar side of the hand, should always prompt consideration of **ulnar-mammary syndrome** and nipple absence or hypoplasia strongly supports this diagnosis. Other signs are abnormal placement of the anus, which may be stenotic, and small male genitalia. Limb malformations, typically of ectrodactyly (split hand/foot), in association with nipple hypoplasia signal **ectrodactyly-ectodermal dysplasia syndrome** (EEC), or a variant thereof, the condition being clinically highly heterogeneous.

Investigations to Consider Isoelectric focusing of transferrin is the best way to detect almost all cases of CDG variants but may not be sensitive in the first few weeks of life until abnormal forms build up. Ulnar-mammary syndrome may be confirmed by *TBX3* gene mutation analysis and EEC clinical variants thereof by *p63* gene mutations.

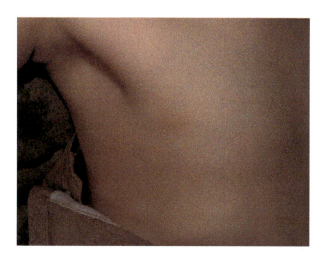

Figure 7.3 A small hypoplastic nipple with little surrounding pigment and an almost complete absence of areola is shown in a patient who presented neonatally with choanal atresia and whose mother had been treated for hyperthyroidism with carbimazole throughout pregnancy.

7.4 Gynecomastia

Recognizing the Sign Excess breast development in male patients must be considered in terms of normal physiologic gynecomastia, which may be observed neonatally and at adolescence. This is generally bilateral and transient. Breast enlargement, resembling gynecomastia, is a feature of obesity. Widely described in adult male populations with hyperthyroidism, hypothyroidism, liver failure, and chronic renal failure, gynecomastia is rare in the prepubertal child.

Establishing a Differential Diagnosis An impression of gynecomastia in a thin baby, particularly if there is a history of intrauterine growth retardation and failure to thrive, may reflect a generalized lipodystrophy of **leprechaunism**. Signs of acanthosis nigricans would support the diagnosis of this autosomal recessive condition. These children are noteworthy for the well-defined appearance of their musculature, the subcutaneous fat being deficient. However, most gynecomastia is a postpubertal phenomenon, in which instance, signs of normal sexual development should be sought. One of the most common causes of gynecomastia is **Klinefelter syndrome** (47, XXY), in which the associated small gonads and penis, long limbs, and, occasionally but not reliably, a history of behavioral or mild developmental concerns may be forthcoming. However, many Klinefelter cases only present in adult life at infertility clinics. Think specifically about **Kallmann syndrome**, especially if there is developmental delay—check the patient for repaired cleft palate or subclinical clefting in the form of bifid uvula. Some Kallman patients may have generalized dry skin from an X chromosome deletion and the observation of mirror movements on neurologic evaluation is very strongly suggestive of this diagnosis. If observed, specific neurologic assessment for anosmia is warranted. The presence of skin lentigines in gynecomastia cases enjoying normal secondary sexual characteristics is important because of the association with silent but potentially devastating atrial myxoma—this autosomal dominant association being known as **Carney complex;** a family history may offer additional diagnostic support. A presentation of emerging gynecomastia in a previously normal nonobese adult man requires careful evaluation of neurologic status of the lower cranial nerves. Any perioral fasciculation, tongue weakness, or swallowing difficulties will strongly suggest the diagnosis of **X-linked spinal muscular atrophy**.

Investigations to Consider Karyotype is indicated to look for the 47, XXY of Klinefelter syndrome. Evaluation of endocrine status is warranted if no other clinical signs prompt a diagnosis. Echocardiography should be conducted for myxomata if lentigines are present. Mutations of the androgen receptor gene are demonstrable in X-linked spinal muscular atrophy (SMA) and of the insulin receptor gene in leprechaunism; deletion of the *Kal1* gene on Xp22 is the most common molecular cause of Kallman syndrome.

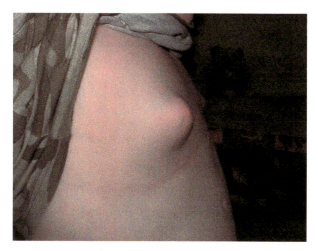

Figure 7.4 Bilateral gynecomastia is demonstrated in this 14-year-old patient referred for evaluation of pubertal delay, who proved to have Kallmann syndrome. The genitalia were very small and anosmia was confirmed on formal testing.

7.5 Sloping Shoulders

Recognizing the Sign Absence of the normal horizontal configuration of the shoulder, due to underlying clavicular bony and/or muscular abnormality, results in shoulders that slope and are almost continuous with the neck.

Establishing a Differential Diagnosis This sign is classically, but not exclusively, seen in the autosomal dominant condition **cleidocranial dysostosis** (CCD). This condition is usually identifiable at birth, the facial features of a high, prominent, bossed forehead often accompanied by very large fontanelles, hypertelorism, and the characteristic absence of well-demarcated shoulders. In later life, the patients demonstrate a facility to voluntarily oppose the shoulders, owing to the hypoplasia of the acromial ends of the clavicles. Good corroborative evidence for the condition in the older patient is found in the teeth, in which delayed loss of deciduous teeth is often followed by an edentulous period before the very delayed eruption of permanent dentition. Abnormally short clavicles and associated neck webbing in some patients with **craniofrontonasal dysplasia** (CFND) give a shoulder configuration similar to CCD. Usually the facial features, with prominent widow's peak and bifid nasal tip, signal the true diagnosis. Despite the frequent coincidental absence of the corpus callosum in CFND patients, intelligence is generally normal. Most patients with branchiootorenal (BOR) syndrome have entirely normal shoulders, but one variant with sloping shoulders, typical of CCD in appearance, is the condition known as **oto-facio-cervical syndrome**. This should be suspected in a child with sloping shoulders who also has deafness. Examine specifically for preauricular pits, branchial cysts, and evidence of underlying renal malformations. Sloping shoulders are occasionally encountered in **Holt-Oram syndrome**, but the diagnosis in this situation will be clear because of associated congenital heart disease, most commonly atrial septal defect (ASD), and more extensive upper limb malformations, which are usually bilateral. Sloping shoulders are also well-recognized within the **Noonan syndrome** phenotype, the diagnosis being suspected by the ptosis, curly hair, and cardiac lesion, most commonly pulmonary stenosis.

Investigations to Consider Radiologic examination of the skeleton in CCD confirms the diagnosis with wormian bones and areas of calvarial thickening in the skull vault, hypoplastic or absent clavicles and scapulae, and hypoplasia of the iliac wings and delayed ossification of the pubis. Mutation of the *CBFA1* gene on chromosome 6 confirms CCD, if there is clinical or radiologic doubt. CFND patients have mutations of the *EFNB1* gene on the X chromosome, while deletion in the region of chromosome 8q around the BOR locus, the gene *EYA1*, is described in oto-facio-cervical syndrome.

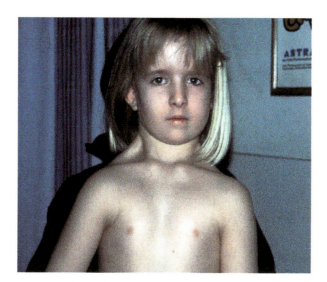

Figure 7.5 This child has the oto-facio-cervical syndrome variant of branchiootorenal syndrome. The sloping shoulders are well demonstrated.

7.6 Small Thorax

Recognizing the Sign A narrow chest can be confirmed by measuring the chest circumference at the nipple level and comparing to normal age-matched values. This is a sign commonly identified antenatally on ultrasound anomaly scans. Whether antenatally or postnatally identified, the length, shape, and radiologic morphology of the long bones will have a major bearing on diagnostic conclusions.

Establishing a Differential Diagnosis It needs to be borne in mind that the age at presentation has a major impact on likely diagnosis—for instance, **thanatophoric dysplasia** (TD) is one of the most common causes of a small thorax ultrasonically, but virtually all these patients die in the immediate neonatal period. In examining a deceased infant with a narrow chest, valuable signs to establish are whether there is clover leaf malformation of the skull (TD), short limbs (TD and camptomelic dysplasia [CD]), blue sclera (osteogenesis imperfecta), postaxial polydactyly (Jeune and Ellis-van Crefeld syndrome), and sexual ambiguity (CD). Ultimately, the diagnosis will depend upon radiologic characteristics, but good clinical documentation can prove invaluable. In the child who has survived the postnatal period but whose chest circumference is narrow, look at the hands for polydactyly and in the mouth for accessory frenula, and examine the heart for a possible ASD, all of which signs betoken the diagnosis of **Ellis-van Crefeld syndrome**. Natal teeth are a very good clue to this diagnosis. Associated findings of short arms and legs, particularly in a baby whose hair is slow to grow, probably represent **McKusick-cartilage-hair hypoplasia syndrome**, which is an important condition to recognize because of the associated susceptibility to varicella infection and defects of cellular immunity, occasionally necessitating bone marrow transplantation. Typically the radiologic changes are of metaphyseal dysplasia, worse at the distal end of the femur. Patients with **Jeune asphyxiating thoracic dystrophy** often do not survive, but if they do, they are at risk of cystic renal changes, cirrhosis, and retinal dystrophy. Small numbers of **Campomelic Dysplasia** cases have survived into adult life and should be suspected in narrow-chested individuals with macrocephaly, hypertelorism, hypotonia, micrognathia, and cleft palate.

Investigations to Consider Full skeletal survey is the cornerstone of diagnosis, irrespective of the age at presentation. Chromosomal sex is a valuable test if there is curvature of the femora in a phenotypic female. 46XY patients with CD undergo sex reversal, sometimes complete, more commonly resulting in genital ambiguity, and karyotype can prompt the true diagnosis. Mutation analysis is available for most of these conditions but is rarely needed for diagnostic purposes, radiology in expert hands usually sufficing.

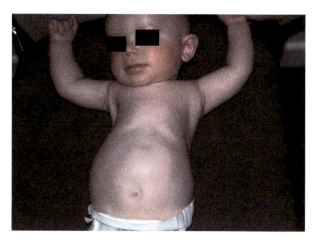

Figure 7.6 Note the narrowing of the thorax in this surviving case of Jeune asphyxiating thoracic dystrophy.

7.7 Pectus Excavatum and Carinatum

Recognizing the Sign The depression of the sternum and costosternal junctions that signals pectus excavatum is easily identified and the rationale for the synonymous term, "funnel chest," clear. The opposite configuration, of sternal protrusion, comprises pectus carinatum. It is worth bearing in mind that these signs may be no more than an isolated finding and not relate to any underlying syndrome.

Establishing a Differential Diagnosis Observe and chart the stature. Is there evidence for excess linear growth, in which case **Marfan syndrome** will need to be considered? Look for arachnodactyly, unusual degrees of joint laxity, lens dislocation (usually upward), and transverse striae in the dorsal thoracic and lumbar regions. The family history may contain clues, specifically of sudden death due to dissecting aneurysm. Long fingers should also prompt clinical enquiry for **Beals syndrome** (congenital contractural arachnodactyly), in which syndrome external ear inspection often discloses a rather crumpled appearance. Careful assessment of the joints, both large and small, may be rewarded by evidence of joint contracture or limitation of full extension. Spinal assessment for scoliosis is an important element of the examination if this condition is being considered. Developmental delay with "marfanoid" characteristics, both of increased linear growth and of arachnodactyly, should cause the observer to consider **homocystinuria** as a possible diagnosis. Lens dislocation (usually downward), restriction of joint movement, kyphoscoliosis, and generalized osteoporosis on x-ray are strong clues to this easily overlooked condition. Pectus excavatum in patients with stature toward the lower end of the normal range warrants a different diagnostic approach. Cardiac examination may reveal a murmur and assessment for **Noonan syndrome** is advised. The classic chest configuration in Noonan cases is of a pectus carinatum above and a pectus excavatum below, but not every case obliges by conforming exactly to the textbook! Ptosis, excess nuchal skin, and low posterior hairline may offer additional corroboration, as may family history and clinical assessment of the parents.

Investigations to Consider Echocardiography is essential if the diagnosis of Marfan syndrome is being considered to assess the aortic root diameter and evaluate for management implications. Prolonged bleeding time is seen in many Noonan cases. Elevated methionine and homocysteine levels on amino acid analysis are suggestive of homocystinuria. *FBN1* mutation analysis is occasionally useful in Marfan syndrome, while mutation of *FBN2* is characteristic of Beals syndrome.

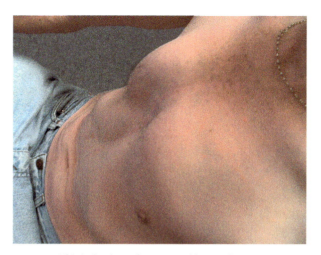

Figure 7.7 This is the chest of a 44-year-old man whose son was sent for clinical genetics assessment for short stature. The boy had undiagnosed Noonan syndrome. The father had had surgery at age 28 for pulmonary stenosis (see the midline sternotomy scar) and his sternal configuration of pectus carinatum superiorly and pectus excavatum inferiorly is classical of Noonan syndrome.

7.8 Scoliosis

Recognizing the Sign Lateral curvature of the spine constitutes scoliosis, which may be isolated or associated with kyphosis, in which posterior angulation of the spine develops. Inspect the spine in the flexed position, and observe any asymmetry in shoulder height, pelvic tilt, and exaggerated lordosis.

Establishing a Differential Diagnosis Scoliosis is an especially difficult problem to assess as a possible clue to a dysmorphic syndrome, being such an etiologically heterogeneous anomaly. Consider the possible causes and assess whether the spinal problem is idiopathic. Any other clinical feature, such as abnormal limb length or developmental delay, should forestall thoughts of an idiopathic basis! Reduced limb length and limitation of joint movement probably indicate that the primary pathology is a **skeletal dysplasia**, which can be a primary disorder or secondary to an underlying biochemical abnormality, such as arises in **mucopolysaccharidoses** and other storage disorders. By contrast, an increase in limb length or excessive joint laxity might be the clinical clue to consider a **connective tissue disorder** as the primary disease process. Accordingly, the clinical examination will focus on the skin for signs of fragility, striae, or excess bruising and the eyes for blue sclera. Specific clinical examination, such as for evidence of lens dislocation in suspected **Marfan syndrome**, may be warranted. Scoliosis is a frequent late childhood complication of those clinical entities described as "associations" on the basis of the frequent nonrandom observation of the anomalies coinciding in individuals. Hence, a history of the neonatal and childhood period may give a clue—a history of cardiac surgery may indicate that the child had **VATER association** (*v*ertebrae, imperforate *a*nus, *t*racheoesophageal fistula, radial +/− *r*enal anomalies) and the scoliosis is an understandable late manifestation of this, hemivertebrae being a frequent finding. Finally, there are specific syndromes of which scoliosis can be a severe complication. **Neurofibromatosis type 1** should be readily identifiable in a scoliotic child by the skin manifestations of café-au-lait patches and axillary freckling. **Coffin-Lowry syndrome** should be considered in boys with a history of developmental delay who present with scoliosis and the rather coarse facial features, full lips, and characteristically puffy fingers sought at examination (Figure 9.9). Finally, the author has seen several cases of **Sotos syndrome**, in whom that diagnosis was missed in early life, present with scoliosis at 5 or 6 years of age. Early developmental concerns, macrocephaly, ruddy cheeks, and large chins are useful clinical indicators of this syndrome.

Investigations to Consider A full skeletal survey is necessary to address whether there is a skeletal dysplasia and possibly identify the underlying condition. Bone age is indicated if Sotos syndrome is suspected—advancement is the general rule.

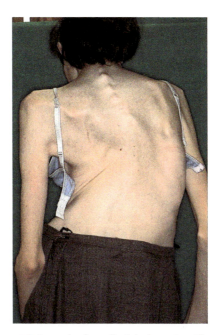

Figure 7.8 Severe kyphoscoliosis is shown in a 15-year-old girl, always considered tall for her age. Examination showed prominent, slightly protruding eyes; multiple skin bruises; and the "criss-cross" pattern of the palms, which is typical of Ehlers-Danlos syndrome type VI—the oculoscoliotic form—in which autosomal recessive condition lysyl hydroxylase deficiency is associated with ocular fragility, blue sclera, prominence of the eyes, and severe vertebral problems. See also Figure 9.18C for the criss-cross pattern.

Chapter 8   The Abdomen and Perineum

8.1 Minor Anomalies of the Umbilicus

Recognizing the Sign The normal position of the umbilicus is at the level of the top of the iliac crests, opposite the third or fourth lumbar vertebra. The umbilicus is extraordinary for its variation, there being no "standard." Minor anomalies, if recognized, can impart diagnostically important information and guide the clinician toward an initially unsuspected diagnosis. In this respect, three particular variations are noteworthy: (1) ovoid depression surrounding a prominent, protruding umbilicus; (2) prominent umbilicus with redundant periumbilical skin; and (3) upward displacement of the umbilicus toward the xiphisternum.

Establishing a Differential Diagnosis Ovoid depression of the tissue immediately surrounding the umbilicus, resulting in a lozenge-shaped depression encircling a slightly prominent umbilicus, is entirely typical of the X-linked short stature condition **Aarskog syndrome**, being very infrequently seen in any other situation. Faced with this observation, the clinical examination will focus on the patient's stature, but also on other clinical features typical of this condition—hypertelorism is usual in such cases and ptosis very common; the hands frequently show mild skin syndactyly and hyperextension of the fingers at the proximal interphalangeal joints. Brachydactyly is usual (Figure 9.7B). Genital examination is important, the penis having a characteristic "shawl" configuration, in which the scrotal folds are inserted above the base of the penis (see 8.7 and Figure 8.7). Family history may support the likely diagnosis, and carrier females may themselves show short stature and brachydactyly. Redundant periumbilical skin around a prominent umbilicus often gets mistaken for a small umbilical hernia and is treated surgically. A history such as this is typical of patients with **Rieger syndrome**, an autosomal dominant condition of hypodontia, anterior segment of the eye malformation, and characteristic failure of involution of the periumbilical skin. A family history of "umbilical hernia" is an excellent pointer toward this diagnosis. Examine the teeth for hypodontia and oligodontia. Cleft palate is an occasional finding. Anterior chamber eye malformations need to be specifically sought by expert ophthalmologic evaluation. Finally, an upwardly displaced umbilicus demands examination for other features of **Robinow syndrome**, this feature being observed in many Robinow patients. A cleft lip, familial short stature, anteverted nares, and micropenis in the male are all strongly supportive of this underlying diagnosis (Figure 2.5A).

Investigations to Consider The diagnosis in all instances is primarily clinical. Skeletal radiology is complementary in Aarskog cases, showing nonspecific metaphyseal dysplasia and bone age delay. Hand radiology in Robinow may show bifid terminal phalanges to the thumbs and halluces. Mutation analysis is available in all instances for clinically doubtful examples.

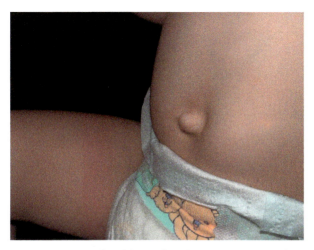

Figure 8.1A A typical umbilicus of Aarskog syndrome in profile, showing the periumbilical depression surrounding the minimally protruding umbilicus. See Figure 2.1A for the facial features of Aarskog syndrome.

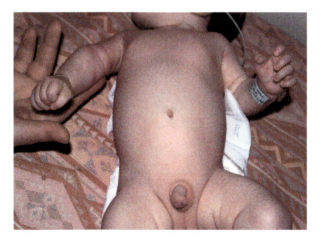

Figure 8.1B A cranially displaced umbilicus is shown. Note also the shawl scrotum (see section 8.7) and the hypoplasia of the scrotum.

8.2　Umbilical Hernia/Omphalocele

Recognizing the Sign This is an easy sign to identify, being a skin-covered protrusion of the umbilicus, due to defective closure of the umbilical ring. In most babies, the umbilical ring closes within the first 2 years of life and persistence beyond this age is associated with a declining rate of spontaneous closure. A large umbilical hernia at birth may be, more correctly, an omphalocele, in which abdominal contents, covered by peritoneum, herniate into the cord.

Establishing a Differential Diagnosis Omphalocele is a well-recognized presentation of **Beckwith-Wiedemann syndrome** (BWS). A history of polyhydramnios, large birth weight, and neonatal hypoglycemia should be sought. Examination should assess for nevus flammeus, macroglossia, ear lobe creases, and punched-out depressions of the helical rim and posterior aspect of the pinna, as well as organomegaly. There is an increased prevalence among babies conceived by assisted reproductive technologies. Long-term surveillance for neoplasms is usual. Other conditions to consider in the newborn period are the trisomies, omphaloceles being well described in **trisomy 21, 18,** and **13**. The distinction of BWS from Down syndrome, in which a clinical impression of macroglossia derives from a somewhat reduced oral cavity volume, should not be taken for granted, proving rather challenging on well-remembered occasions in the delivery ward! Macroglossia is a rarely recognized feature of several forms of **Ehlers-Danlos syndrome** (EDS), in which disorders there is a propensity to neonatal inguinal hernias developing and, although admittedly rare, the author has seen three cases of EDS diagnosed neonatally as BWS. Neonatal umbilical hernia is well recognized in **congenital hypothyroidism,** which should be identified by Guthrie screening. Likewise, persisting umbilical hernia in a child whose development is starting to give cause for concern may be the presentation of **mucopolysaccharidosis** (MPS) I and II. Examination for the characteristic corneal clouding is advised. By contrast, **Sanfilippo syndrome**, MCP III, does not show corneal clouding and the presentation is often at age 3 or 4 years, with persisting umbilical hernia or hernia that may have been operated upon, persistent diarrhea, progressively unruly behavior, and, identifiable only by reviewing old photographs, coarsening of the facies.

Investigations to Consider Molecular testing for BWS is very complex but mutation of the *CDKN1C* gene is particularly common among cases presenting with omphalocele. Do basic karyotype if in clinical doubt about trisomy. Urinary screen for MCP will identify excess glycosaminoglycan (GAG) in MCP I and II, but diagnosis of type III can be elusive and the best screening test is not urinary GAG but vacuolated lymphocytes on peripheral blood smear.

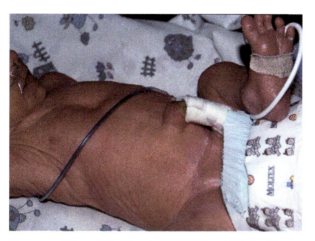

Figure 8.2A The umbilical hernia in this baby with Beckwith-Wiedemann syndrome is a strong clue to the diagnosis. The macroglossia can just be seen.

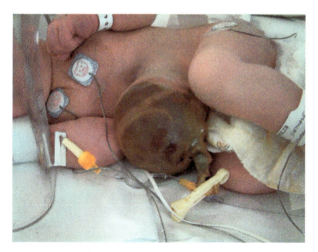

Figure 8.2B A typical example of omphalocoele in another patient with Beckwith-Wiedemann syndrome. (Courtesy of Dr. M. Thomas.)

8.3 Inguinal Hernia

Recognizing the Sign Tenfold more common among male than female children, widening of the external inguinal ring facilitates the herniation of a loop of bowel into the inguinal canal and scrotum. The resultant hernia is easily seen on inspection. Ten percent are bilateral.

Establishing a Differential Diagnosis Among phenotypic females, bilaterality, being rare, should arouse suspicion. Many **androgen insensitivity** cases present with this pattern and careful internal examination ultrasonically and at laparotomy confirms the diagnosis—but only if the examining clinician is alive to the likely diagnosis. Of course, most inguinal hernias are nonsyndromic, especially if related to **prematurity**. However, several syndromes have an increased prevalence of hernia. Foremost among these are the **mucopolysaccharidoses** and a low threshold for investigation of these disorders in children with inguinal hernia in the first few months of life is strongly advised, even if corneal clouding and more "classical" syndromic signs have not yet appeared. The hernia may herald the onset of problems retrospectively identifiable as MCP related. The second category of syndrome to bear in mind are **connective tissue disorders** such as Marfan, Ehlers-Danlos (EDS) complex, and cutis laxa syndromes. Their differentiation may require expert clinical and/or laboratory assistance but signs of excess skin, skin fragility, hypermobility of joints, and thin skin in which veins are easily seen are all strong clues to this group of conditions. Since many of these disorders are dominant, details of the family history may not only confirm the likely diagnosis, but also specify one disorder above others. Unique clinical features, such as the presence of nasal papillomata in Costello syndrome cases, facilitate the differentiation of particular disorders from clinically overlapping entities. Finally, the examiner needs to be aware of a few individual syndromes associated with inguinal hernia. Careful assessment for **Williams syndrome** is advised—was there hypercalcemia neonatally? Is there a cardiac murmur? Do the eyes have a stellate iris pattern? Is there flare of the eyebrow medially? In the older child, are there developmental concerns? Compare the facial features with early photographs and assess for any slight coarsening. If there is short stature, think specifically of **Aarskog syndrome** and look for shawl scrotum as a likely clue to diagnosis.

Investigations to Consider Urinary GAG and skeletal radiology are indicated to assess for MCP. Karyotype in females is warranted to exclude androgen insensitivity. Urinary pyridinoline cross-links for EDS VI and serum tenascin X for EDS-like syndromes. Fluorescence in situ hybridization (FISH) of *ELN* is indicated for Williams syndrome. Molecular diagnosis for many variants of connective tissue disorders is available, but suspecting the diagnosis is primarily a clinical exercise.

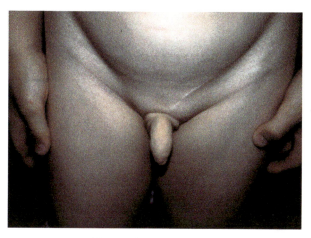

Figure 8.3 Repaired left-sided inguinal hernia is seen in this boy with Aarskog syndrome. Note the shawl scrotum hinting directly at the underlying syndrome diagnosis.

8.4 Small Penis/Micropenis

Recognizing the Sign A subjective impression of a small penis should be confirmed by measurement and charting against normal values. The measurement is taken from the pubic bone to the tip of the glans.

Establishing a Differential Diagnosis Pure **endocrine causes** will generally not result in associated malformations, so the examination needs to focus on syndromes that are associated with micropenis. The iris may show a coloboma, or a cardiac murmur may be heard, which should lead to an evaluation of the external ear for possible overfolding of the helix, all of which may be indicative of **CHARGE association** (*c*oloboma, *h*eart, *a*tresia choana, *r*etarded growth, *g*enital abnormalities, *e*ar malformations). Unilateral choanal atresia may be present but unrecognized, bilaterality usually presenting early. Floppiness in the newborn with micropenis, especially in the presence of a need for assisted feeding and a poor suck, should prompt concern for **Prader-Willi syndrome**. In the older case, the almond-shaped eyes, narrow hands, and straight ulnar border will clinically suggest the diagnosis, but the characteristic eating behavioral disorder will be the main clue after the first 2 years. Careful evaluation of the hands and feet may show postaxial "nubbins"—vestigial polydactyly, which frequently signifies **Bardet-Biedl syndrome**. Developmental delay, emerging obesity, and a reduced ability to concentrate urine will characterize the natural history of this autosomal recessive disorder, which is associated with retinal dystrophy but usually not before the second decade of life. **Klinefelter syndrome** must be considered, especially in patients who fail to enter puberty. Tall stature is usual and gynecomastia a valuable clue, if present. Breast abnormality is likewise the prompt for suspecting cases of **ulnar-mammary syndrome**, with gynecomastia but, more likely, breast hypoplasia being common. Evaluate the hands for evidence of ulnar defects, missing fingers, or hypoplasia. Boys with **Robinow syndrome** (Figure 2.5A) as the basis of their micropenis will have the typical facial features of hypertelorism and anteverted nares and the umbilicus may be displaced cranially, while cleft palate or lip associated with micropenis should prompt concern for **Kallmann syndrome**, in which developmental delay is common; mirror movements are an excellent clinical clue and anosmia an almost invariable feature.

Investigations to Consider Most patients with CHARGE have semicircle canal aplasia/hypoplasia and computed tomography (CT) of the petrous temporal bones can secure the diagnosis in clinically doubtful situations. Mutation of the *CHD7* gene is established in CHARGE. Paternal 15q deletion studies for Prader-Willi syndrome sometimes need further molecular supplementation, while basic karyotype will confirm 47,XXY in Klinefelter cases. Deletion of the *KAL1* gene is the commonest cause of Kallman syndrome but the molecular diagnosis of Bardet-Biedl syndrome remains extremely complex due to the sheer number of genes involved.

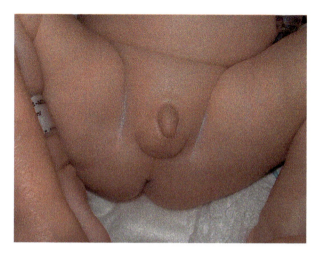

Figure 8.4 Micropenis is demonstrated in a newborn whose presentation was with a heart murmur due to a ventricular septal defect (VSD). Further examination showed bilateral retinal colobomata, hypoplastic semicircular canals, and unilateral choanal atresia. The diagnosis was CHARGE association.

8.5 Ambiguous Genitalia

Recognizing the Sign The appearance of the external genitalia manifests elements of both male and female development.

Establishing a Differential Diagnosis The single most common cause is **21α-hydroxylase deficiency**, an autosomal recessive nonsyndromic enzymatic deficiency requiring investigation of the adrenal gland for possible salt-losing crisis. This and other biochemical causes of a nonsyndromic nature, such as **androgen insensitivity,** are not considered further here. Primary among the clinician's concerns must be to establish whether the baby has other malformations or clinical clues to a syndromic diagnosis. Examine the eyes—specifically, query whether there is aniridia. Your concern is for **WAGR** (*W*ilms tumor, *a*niridia, *g*enital anomalies, *r*etardation) syndrome due to deletion of the *WT1* gene on chromosome 11p13. A related condition to also consider is **Drash syndrome**, in which early-onset hypertension, proteinuria, and nephropathy develop in children with 46XY genotype whose genitalia are female or ambiguous and is due to a *WT1* gene mutation. Examine the limbs; 2/3 syndactyly of the toes is a good clue to **Smith-Lemli-Opitz (S-L-O) syndrome** and if present, look for facial features of bitemporal narrowing and anteversion of the nostrils. Limitation of extension at the joints, particularly the elbow, with evidence of craniosynostosis should prompt consideration of **Antley-Bixler syndrome**. This condition can be mimicked fairly exactly by maternal ingestion of Fluconazole during pregnancy. Exstrophy of the bladder, omphalocele, and anal agenesis result in ambiguous or grossly abnormal genitalia as part of a series of well-recognized patterns of associated malformation but of unknown basis, such as **urorectal septum defects** and **OEIS** (*o*mphalocele, *e*xstrophy of bladder, *i*mperforate anus, and *s*acral anomalies). Ambiguous genitalia can be the first clinically recognizable feature of **α-thalassemia mental retardation, X-linked** (ATRX), so a family history of male mental retardation should not be discounted as irrelevant. Assess the face for coarseness, especially around the upper lip, while small teeth and depressed nasal bridge are good facial clues in a slightly older age group (see Figure 1.6C).

Investigations to Consider Karyotype is indicated to establish the chromosomal sex. Ambiguous genitalia are a reported feature of several chromosomal abnormalities and an abnormal karyotype may itself offer adequate explanation of the phenotype. Specifically request 11p FISH studies if WAGR is suspected. *WT1* mutation analysis is indicated for Drash syndrome, but proteinuria should be consistently present to justify this investigation. Serum cholesterol and 7-dehydrocholesterol are needed to diagnose S-L-O. Though mutation analysis is available for ATRX syndrome, HbH inclusion bodies on staining with freshly constituted brilliant cresyl blue are a very good screening test, positive in 90% of cases.

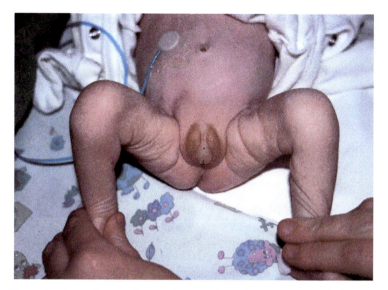

Figure 8.5 A complex translocation between three chromosomes was the basis of the ambiguous genitalia in this baby who had an XY karyotype.

8.6 Hypospadias

Recognizing the Sign The condition is easily recognized provided it is looked for, the urethral meatus being situated on the ventral surface of the penis and proximal to the glans penis.

Establishing a Differential Diagnosis Hypospadias is a relatively common malformation, many cases being isolated nonsyndromic events. Assessment of the kidneys and urinary tract is mandatory in all. Likewise, there are hundreds of syndromes in which hypospadias is described but in many, Fraser syndrome representing a case in point, with cryptophthalmos being the primary feature the clinician will address, the hypospadias is cast in a supporting role, in diagnostic terms. The purpose here is to highlight conditions that ought to be considered if there is a clinical finding of hypospadias. Primary among these are **Smith-Lemli-Opitz (S-L-O) syndrome**, an autosomal recessive condition in which the observation of 2/3 syndactyly of the toes, partial or complete, strongly supports the need for biochemical investigation. Bitemporal narrowing, ptosis, and evidence of developmental delay are characteristic, though not reliably present. Holoprosencephaly is an occasional presentation of S-L-O, so be aware of this diagnosis in the holoprosencephalic infant with hypospadias. Hypertelorism should be noted, as it is a cardinal feature of **Opitz G syndrome**, an X-linked condition associated with hypospadias and swallowing difficulties, sometimes with laryngeal cleft. Laryngoscopic examination is advised. Evaluate the mother, as carriers often show mild degrees of hypertelorism and such observations can clench a diagnosis in difficult circumstances, as can a family history. An ectopic or stenotic anus can constitute part of the Opitz G syndrome spectrum, but may also be significant of **Townes-Brocks syndrome** (T-BS) in a hypospadias presentation. Apart from lacking the hypertelorism of Opitz G, the presence of overfolded ears, preauricular pits, and deafness betray the true syndrome diagnosis of T-BS. Already discussed under ambiguous genitalia (section 8.5), assessment for **WAGR** is warranted likewise in hypospadias, while a rare autosomal recessive condition, easily missed and which frequently presents with hypospadias, is that of **Schinzel-Giedion syndrome**. Generalized hirsutism, fleshy earlobes, and narrow and deep-set nails are features that substantiate this diagnosis, but the main facial features that dysmorphologists agree on are bitemporal narrowing and an infraorbital groove, much as described in fetal valproate syndrome.

Investigations to Consider Karyotype, including 11p FISH studies, is indicated for WAGR. Cholesterol and 7-dehydrocholesterol are warranted for S-L-O. *MID1* mutation is confirmed in many cases of Opitz G syndrome. T-BS is a clinical diagnosis, but mutation analysis of *SALL1* confirms or refutes doubtful cases. The best test for Schinzel-Giedion syndrome is skull x-ray, which typically shows an occipital "gap" in ossification due to synchondrosis.

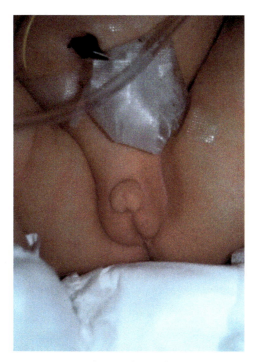

Figure 8.6 Severe hypospadias is demonstrated in a patient with Smith-Lemli-Opitz syndrome. Apart from the genital malformation, the main clinical clue was partial 2/3 syndactyly of the feet.

8.7   Shawl Scrotum and Penoscrotal Transposition

Recognizing the Sign A shawl scrotum gives the appearance of a gothic arch-shaped fold of skin above the base of the penis. Essentially, the genital tubercle, whence the penis derives, has been displaced caudally to a minor degree. In more severe displacement, the penis emerges from the scrotal sac and, at the most extreme end of the spectrum, the penis and scrotum are transposed.

Establishing a Differential Diagnosis The initial impression on inspection often is of micropenis, which should be measured and charted against standard norms. Usually the penis is of normal size on objective assessment. Shawl scrotum is one of the cardinal diagnostic features of **Aarskog syndrome**, an X-linked condition of short stature, delayed bone age, and mild developmental delay in many affected individuals. The facial features are distinctive, particularly the hypertelorism, widow's peak, and high forehead (Figure 2.1A). Look out for the umbilicus, which is often displaced cranially and also shows a characteristic lozenge-shaped depression around the umbilicus (section 8.1 and Figure 8.1A). Many of these patients are chance diagnoses, identified when they present for inguinal hernia repair. The hands show brachydactyly, often with clinodactyly and a mild degree of syndactyly (Figure 9.7B). Typically there is hyperextension of the proximal interphalangeal joints on extension. The family history and review of photographs of family occasions may reveal several other affected individuals. Transposition of the penis and scrotum is extremely uncommon but is seen occasionally in association with anal anomalies in **urorectal septal defects sequence**, where septation of the primitive cloaca is abnormal. Clinical presentations include absence of the penis, ambiguous genitalia, a "smooth" perineum, common exits for anal and urethral channels, in addition to renal malformations. All cases are sporadic and are frequently complicated by congenital heart disease.

Investigations to Consider Skeletal radiology in Aarskog syndrome will show delayed bone age; short limbs, predominantly rhizomelic in character; and mild metaphyseal dysplasia. Mutation analysis of the *FGD1* locus on Xp11.21 confirms mutations in affected individuals if the clinical diagnosis is in doubt. Karyotype and renal tract evaluation are worth undertaking in penoscrotal transposition.

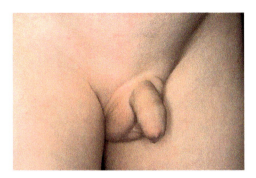

Figure 8.7A A typical shawl scrotum configuration is shown in this patient with Aarskog syndrome. This is the same patient as in Figure 9.7B. See Figure 2.1A for the facial features of Aarskog syndrome.

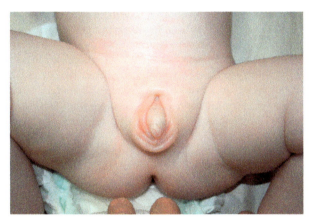

Figure 8.7B An even more pronounced instance of shawl scrotum is shown in a boy without a diagnosis.

8.8 Anal Atresia, Anal Stenosis, and Anterior Displacement of the Anus

Recognizing the Sign Inspect the perineum. Surface signs of fistula on the perineum or to the vulva should be sought. The anus may be present but be almost continuous with the vagina, with little clear separation. In males, hypospadias and bifid scrotum may be observed.

Establishing a Differential Diagnosis The family history will usually identify the autosomal dominant condition **Currarino syndrome**, in which anal malformations and/or chronic childhood constipation may be the presenting feature. Be aware of the possibility of cerebrospinal fistula, and a history of deaths from *Escherichia coli* meningitis in the family should not be discounted as irrelevant. In the event of a normal family history, assess the palate. Has there been nasal regurgitation during feeding, or is there a cleft? Anal stenosis is an overlooked aspect of **velo-cardio-facial** (VCF) syndrome, so do listen to the heart and look for asymmetric crying facies. **Cat-eye syndrome**, due to mosaic trisomy 22, is another chromosomal cause of anal stenosis/displacement. Preauricular tags and pits, cardiac defects, and coloboma of the iris comprise the full clinical spectrum, but the diagnosis can be especially elusive in the absence of coloboma and is made only by heightened clinical awareness and diligent investigation. Cat-eye syndrome cases can manifest significant clinical overlap with **Townes-Brocks syndrome** (T-BS), and ear and anal malformations are common to both these conditions. However, triphalangeal thumbs and distal thumb deviation offer a specific diagnostic clue to T-BS, if present, but the distinction between these two disorders is occasionally beyond clinical resolution. **VATER association** (*v*ertebrae, imperforate *a*nus, *t*racheo*œ*sophageal fistula, *r*adial +/– renal anomalies) is well known, comprising the association of vertebral, anal, tracheoesophageal, and radial malformations in varying degrees. Less well recognized but equally associated with anal malformations is **Pallister-Hall syndrome** (P-HS), in which a presentation of an anal malformation can mask underlying hypopituitarism and a hypothalamic hamartoblastoma. Polydactyly, either postaxial or mesoaxial (an extra middle finger), should alert the clinician to this important diagnosis. Hypertelorism and hypospadias will signify **Opitz G syndrome** and the need for formal assessment for laryngeal cleft.

Investigations to Consider Sacral radiology shows a characteristic "crescent" shape in 75% of Currarino cases. Magnetic resonance imaging (MRI) scan of the sacrum may show presacral mass. Mutation of the *HLXB9* gene is possible for doubtful or sporadic cases. Karyotype in anal malformations needs to focus on 22q11 FISH; 7qter for tiny deletions and for marker chromosome 22, often lost in blood and fibroblast studies may be needed for diagnosis. *SALLI* mutation confirms T-BS and *GLI3* mutation establishes P-HS.

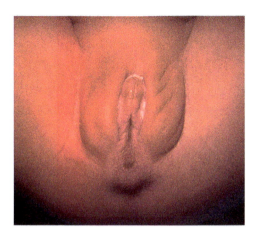

Figure 8.8A The anterior placement of the anus in this example has displaced the anal opening right next to the vestibule. (Courtesy of Professor Prem Puri.)

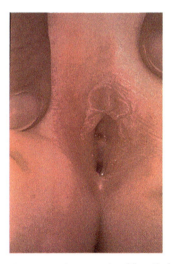

Figure 8.8B An example of "vestibular anus" is shown, in which the anal opening is within the vestibule, the vagina and anus sharing a common wall for about 3 cm. (Courtesy of Professor Prem Puri.)

8.9 Caudal Appendage

Recognizing the Sign A tail is attached to the lumbar or coccygeal region in the midline.

Establishing a Differential Diagnosis Most such instances comprise non-bony appendages of fat, muscle, nerve, and blood vessels and arise as rare sporadic anomalies without syndromic associations. However, in the same way that a hairy patch, dimple, lipoma, or sinus over the lower spine can signify underlying diastematomyelia, a caudal appendage should be viewed as potentially signifying an underlying anomaly and the spinal cord of such individuals merits investigation. There are specific syndromic associations—for instance, with severe forms of **craniosynostosis** and in cases of Crouzon and Pfeiffer syndromes, the patient's abnormal cranial morphology will be the first clinical issue to command attention. The finding of caudal appendage should be recognized as comprising an element of the same underlying genetic disorder and not a distinct pathology. The observation of caudal appendage in a baby who was otherwise "normal" should prompt re-evaluation, as there are a few well-recognized syndromes to which this sign can be a clue. Relook at the face for signs of **Pallister-Killian syndrome**, particularly hypertelorism, coarse features, and temporal balding. Is there evidence for developmental delay? Assess the eyes and particularly the shape of the palpebral fissure for possible **Kabuki syndrome**—you are looking for an elongated fissure, often best recognized by seeing blood vessels in the lateral margin of the fissure (Figure 3.15B). Observe also for ectropion of the lower eyelid and blue sclerae. Lip pits, if present, should be noted and fetal finger pads, are solid, though subtle, clues to this elusive clinical diagnosis. In a boy with large birth weight, think of **Simpson-Golabi-Behmel (S-G-B) syndrome** and assess for cleft palate, deep midline tongue and lower lip groove, congenital heart disease, hypospadias, and polydactyly, or evidence of surgically resected polydactyly. Since this is X-linked, the family history and observation of other family members may betray important diagnostic clues.

Investigations to Consider MRI of the spine is indicated for evidence of cord tethering. In association with craniosynostosis, a syndromic diagnosis can be reached clinically and molecular confirmation of mutations at *FGFR1/FGFR2/FGFR3* loci can be undertaken, dependant on the particular phenotype. Skin karyotype is necessary to identify the tetrasomy 12p of Pallister-Killian syndrome, while mutation analysis of *GPC3* on Xq will confirm suspected cases of S-G-B syndrome.

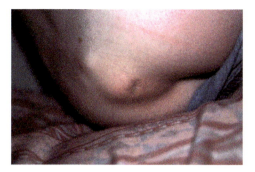

Figure 8.9A A caudal appendage is shown in this 13-year-old boy who presented with lower limb spasticity and increasing clumsiness. Magnetic resonance imaging scan confirmed cord tethering. His parents recalled that this had always been present—specifically, they commented that as a baby it was painful to sit him on their knee for any small period as his appendage caused them such discomfort.

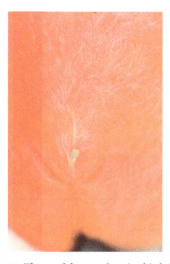

Figure 8.9B The caudal appendage in this baby, born at 35 weeks gestation and who perished within a few days, was a strong clue to the underlying diagnosis of Pallister-Killian syndrome, which fibroblast karyotype confirmed.

Chapter 9   **The Hands**

9.1 Postaxial Polydactyly

Recognizing the Sign An extra digit is present on the ulnar side of the hand. This can be subtle and consist of no more than a small projection of tissue, usually between the metacarpophalangeal and proximal interphalangeal creases.

Establishing a Differential Diagnosis This is one of the most common of all congenital anomalies and can run in families as a harmless autosomal dominant trait. In the event of a normal family history, syndromic consideration must be addressed. Remember to assess for **Patau syndrome** (trisomy 13). The presence of cleft lip and/or a cardiac murmur will increase your concerns that this is the real diagnosis. A cardiac murmur might also make you think about **Ellis-van Creveld syndrome** (EvC). To substantiate this diagnosis, look in the mouth for multiple oral frenula. The additional observation of natal teeth is very strong evidence for this condition. The nails may be small and deep set and the thorax narrow. A narrow thorax is the defining clinical characteristic of **Jeune asphyxiating thoracic dystrophy**, most cases of which expire shortly after birth and many of whom also have a postaxial polydactyly. Survivors can develop a nephronophthisis and retinal dystrophy. The polydactyly of **Meckel-Gruber syndrome**, a lethal autosomal recessive condition, is usually noted by way of confirming the diagnosis in a patient presenting with a Potter-type history of oligohydramnios, encephalocele, and grossly enlarged cystic kidneys. Skull malformation, suggestive of craniosynostosis, is the best prompt to **Carpenter syndrome**, in which postaxial polydactyly of the hand is associated with syndactyly and short fingers. Duplication of the hallux is an unreliable clinical sign in the feet, being absent in several reported cases. Postaxial polydactyly is often the only clue to **Bardet-Biedl syndrome** (BBS) at the time of birth. Emerging obesity in the first year of life, despite normal appetite, consolidates the clinical concerns. The signature retinal dystrophy is often a phenomenon of the second decade and therefore not diagnostically reliable in the young. Hypogenitalism is universal in males and should be sought clinically to support the likely diagnosis in obese males with polydactyly.

Investigations to Consider A basic karyotype will demonstrate the additional chromosome 13 in Patau syndrome. Skeletal radiology in E-vC and Jeune syndromes both show a hook-like downward projection from the medial and lateral acetabular margins, in addition to narrow thorax. Electroretinography (ERG) is often helpful in establishing the diagnosis in BBS before retinal signs become clinically apparent. BBS mutations are known in several genes but have not been a diagnostically valuable investigation in individual cases.

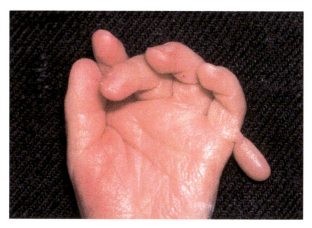

Figure 9.1A Classic postaxial polydactyly in a case of autosomal dominant nonsyndromic familial postaxial polydactyly, the baby's father and grandmother having had the same anomaly.

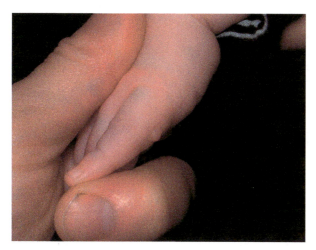

Figure 9.1B Postaxial polydactyly in a 1-year-old boy referred to clinic because of emerging concerns with respect to development. His weight was increased, being above the 97th percentile, and with this history, the polydactyly and hypogenitalism pointed toward a diagnosis of Bardet-Biedl syndrome.

9.2 Preaxial Polydactyly/Thumb Duplication

Recognizing the Sign This uncommon phenomenon is characterized by complete or partial reduplication of a normal biphalangeal thumb. Clinically, you may see a second thumb adjacent to the normal, but if the duplication is confined to the distal phalanx, the clinical presentation may be of a broad nail on the thumb, perhaps with a central line of fusion between the two nails forming the fused nail. It is an uncommon clinical sign.

Establishing a Differential Diagnosis Examine both hands and feet for other evidence of polydactyly, syndactyly, or developmental malformation of the digits. Family history may offer clues, in that rare pedigrees are known with this malformation segregating in autosomal dominant manner. Teratogenic influences should be sought, reduplication, more typically involving the hallux but occasionally of the thumb, being described in maternal diabetes. Assuming that the thumb malformation is the sole sign, assess for **Robinow syndrome**, in which this specific feature is well described. Look at the face for hypertelorism, anteverted nares, and evidence of cleft lip (Figure 2.5A). During infancy, gum hypertrophy is an especially good clue to this diagnosis. The umbilicus may be shifted toward the xiphisternum and males will show micropenis. Assess the ears. Simple, cup-shaped ears are suggestive of **lacrimo-auriculo-dento-digital (LADD) syndrome**, in which deafness, thumb reduplication, and hypodontia occur with nasolacrimal duct obstruction and consequent epiphora. Parents may volunteer that the child never sheds tears on crying—a very good pointer to the diagnosis. Although thumb reduplication is not the most typical hand malformation in **Townes-Brocks syndrome** (T-BS), triphalangeal thumbs being more often encountered clinically, this condition may be the correct diagnosis in the deaf patient with anal malformations, lifelong constipation, and lop ears, perhaps with preauricular pits or skin tags. Careful evaluation of external eye movements is valuable. The observation of a Duane phenomenon, a unilateral sixth nerve palsy with contralateral enophthalmos, strongly suggests that the thumb duplication is the presenting feature of **acro-reno-ocular (ARO) syndrome**, in which deafness and urinary tract anomalies are common. A congenital anemia, especially if associated with cleft lip/palate and the thumb anomaly, urges that the plausible diagnosis of **Blackfan-Diamond syndrome** be considered.

Investigations to Consider Most of the conditions alluded to are clinical diagnoses. Audiologic evaluation is obviously important in LADD, T-BS, and acrorenoocular syndromes. Ophthalmic evaluation is appropriate for possible chorioretinal colobomata in ARO. Mutation analysis of *SALL1* identifies mutations in T-BS and those in the related gene *SALL4* confirm ARO if there is clinical doubt. There is a high risk of renal failure among T-BS cases, so longitudinal renal biochemistry assessment is advisable. Hematologic characterization of anemia will assist identification of Blackfan-Diamond cases.

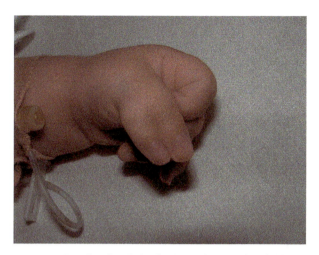

Figure 9.2 Complete thumb duplication is shown in this child with a provisionally unique syndrome.

9.3 Syndactyly of the Fingers

Recognizing the Sign Syndactyly refers to partial or complete fusion between the fingers, which can be osseous or involve the skin only. The interdigital web between fingers 2 and 3 lies at the same level as that between fingers 3 and 4, and any advance in the position of the web signifies cutaneous syndactyly of that web space.

Establishing a Differential Diagnosis Complete syndactyly, often involving the thumb, is typical of **Apert syndrome**, the appearance being termed "mitten hand" malformation. The accompanying skull and facial malformations with eye prominence, beaked nose, and high, turret-shaped skull are easily recognizable. Careful oral examination is warranted, the palate frequently being cleft. Cutaneous syndactyly involving fingers 3 and 4 in a low-birth-weight infant may be the best clinical clue to **triploidy** or diploid/triploid mosaicism. Other clinically recognizable conditions in which syndactyly may be the presenting clinical feature are **Poland anomaly** and **Moebius syndrome**. Accordingly, chest examination for asymmetry of muscle is warranted in the former and cranial nerve evaluation, most particularly of sixth and seventh nerves, in the latter; the examiner is advised to be aware that a small number of cases can have features of both conditions, the Moebius-Poland phenomenon. A specific appearance of syndactyly of fingers 3/4/5 should raise the possibility of **Timothy syndrome**, in which long QT syndrome and a high propensity to arrhythmias and sudden death apply. This same pattern of syndactyly is also seen in **oculo-dento-digital (ODD) syndrome**, the diagnosis being prompted by the hypotelorism, small nose, and enamel hypoplasia (Figure 2.2). Though poorly understood, spasticity of the lower limbs is commonly observed in affected individuals. The most common form of syndactyly is familial, involving fingers 3/4 and toes 2/3, so parental assessment in an infant with syndactyly may exclude syndromic concerns. In association with plagiocephaly, or unusual skull shape, syndactyly is often observed in **Saethre-Chotzen syndrome**. Being autosomal dominant, parental examination may also reveal forehead flattening or other features of craniosynostosis. Ptosis, frontalis overactivity, and prominence of the horizontal ear crus are other valuable clinical signs in securing this diagnosis.

Investigations to Consider Karyotype will establish triploidy (69 chromosomes). Electrocardiography (ECG) and specifically QT-interval evaluation is indicated if Timothy syndrome is being considered. *CACNA1C* gene mutation is established in all cases. Apert syndrome constitutes a clinical diagnosis. *FGFR2* mutation is present in all affected individuals. ODD is caused by *GJA1* mutation. Magnetic resonance imaging (MRI) examination has shown white matter changes in some ODD affected individuals with spasticity. Mutations of the *TWIST* locus on 7p are demonstrable in cases of Saethre-Chotzen syndrome.

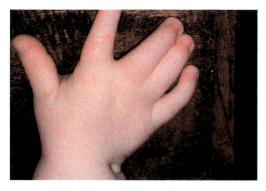

Figure 9.3A Complete syndactyly of fingers 3 and 4 is shown in a patient with triploidy.

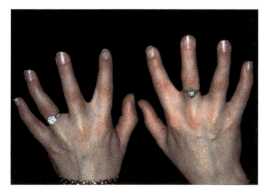

Figure 9.3B The hands shown are of a 24-year-old woman who has Saethre-Chotzen syndrome. Note the bilateral, symmetric cutaneous syndactyly of fingers 2 and 3.

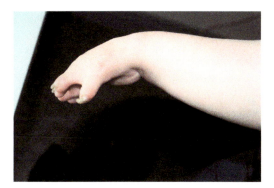

Figure 9.3C Symbrachydactyly associated with Poland anomaly is demonstrated in an adult female patient. In addition to the finger fusion, the digits are short, hence the descriptive term "symbrachydactyly"

9.4　Clinodactyly of the Fingers

Recognizing the Sign This term refers to deflection of one or more fingers medially or laterally. The most common presentation is of medial deviation of the fifth finger due to hypoplasia of the middle phalanx. A good clinical barometer of clinodactyly is to look at the flexion creases of the interphalangeal joints, which slope toward one another in clinodactyly rather than pursuing parallel courses, as is the norm.

Establishing a Differential Diagnosis Clinodactyly is common and frequently familial. Parental evaluation may dissipate syndromic concerns. Alternatively, a form of autosomal dominant brachydactyly may be established and the clinodactyly thus explained. Clinodactyly, especially of the fifth finger, is common, and this minor anomaly simply heightens the awareness of the examiner for other similar signs of abnormal development. Hence, 60% of **Down syndrome** cases will have fifth finger clinodactyly, but the clinical diagnosis of Down syndrome will rest on the presence of other characteristic signs. Likewise, clinodactyly is a nonspecific finding in several chromosomal deletion and duplication syndromes beyond clinical recognition and reliant for determination on karyotypic analysis. However, several short stature syndromes are associated with clinodactyly—in **Russell-Silver syndrome**, the first clue to diagnosis may be the low birth weight and length but relatively normal head circumference. Café-au-lait skin patches often emerge in time. Careful evaluation for asymmetry of the limbs is useful, asymmetry being an associated feature, but absence of limb asymmetry in an otherwise typical Russell-Silver presentation is characteristic of a subgroup of children whose short stature may be due to **disomy of chromosome 7**. Clinodactyly is also common in **Aarskog syndrome,** in which an X-linked history of short stature should be sought. Look for other characteristic findings of hypertelorism, shawl scrotum, and periumbilical depression (Figures 8.1 and 8.7). In the older child referred for developmental concerns, clinodactyly is a good pointer toward **tricho-rhino-phalangeal (TRP) syndrome** (Figures 2.4 and 12.5). On questioning it will be established that the hair is fine, growing poorly in the frontotemporal regions, while evaluation of the nose will often show a bulbous tip. There may be prominent interphalangeal joints with slight deviation of the phalanges causing clinodactyly of other fingers.

Investigations to Consider Karyotype is indicated if trisomy 21 is suspected or clinical signs warrant exclusion of other chromosomal conditions. Disomy 7 studies in symmetric short stature but with a clinical resemblance to Russell-Silver syndrome require parental DNA samples in addition to that of the patient. Hand x-rays may show cone-shaped epiphyses in TRP syndrome and exostoses are sometimes seen on long bones. Deletion of chromosome 8q should be sought if TRP is suspected.

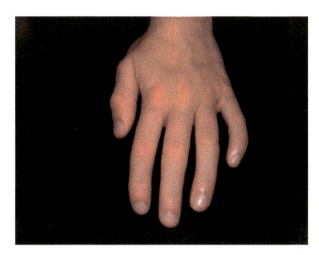

Figure 9.4 Clinodactyly of the fifth finger is shown in this patient with an unknown syndrome of developmental delay. Note also the somewhat small nails of the second and third fingers.

9.5 Arachnodactyly of the Fingers

Recognizing the Sign This description refers to long, thin fingers.

Establishing a Differential Diagnosis Measure the height of the patient and assess the skeletal features clinically. The major concern is to establish whether the patient may have **Marfan syndrome** (MS). Excess joint laxity, pectus carinatum or excavatum, scoliosis, reduced upper-to-lower segment height ratio, and the ability to protrude the thumb below the ulnar border of the enclosed fist are all features that strongly support a likely diagnosis of Marfan syndrome. A positive family history, if procured, can be confirmatory. Ocular evaluation for lens dislocation, skin examination for striae, evidence of hernia repair, and cardiac evaluation for aortic root dilatation or mitral valve prolapse should be undertaken. The misdiagnosis of Marfan syndrome, both diagnosis missed and cases wrongly identified, represents the most common cause of referral to the author's clinic. A common error arises with respect to lens dislocation, often absent if evaluated in the newborn period and assumed therefore to be normal. This feature can develop later, and serial ophthalmic re-evaluation is diagnostically useful in cases where the diagnosis remains in doubt. The closely related condition of **Beals contractural arachnodactyly** usually shows camptodactyly of the fingers and joint contractures of the knees. An unusual "crumpled" appearance to the ear should be sought, the helix being flattened superiorly, and confirms the diagnosis, which is not associated with aortic root weakness. **Homocystinuria** mimics the skeletal features of Marfan syndrome and characteristic downward lens dislocation may not occur until the age of 10 years. Mild developmental delay, the absence of cardiac findings, and a history of seizures or evidence of spasticity clinically represent the best clinical parameters for distinction from MS. A malar flush is often observed. Occasionally **Stickler syndrome** patients demonstrate arachnodactyly. The family history of myopia and/or retinal detachment, cleft palate and micrognathia, and early-onset osteoarthritis will usually serve as a good clinical basis for distinction from MS. The presence of a flat malar region and depressed nasal bridge in a patient should alert the examiner to the likely diagnosis and avert the misdiagnosis of MS.

Investigations to Consider Echocardiography and specific evaluation of aortic root diameter is mandatory if MS is being considered, having both diagnostic and management value. *FBN1* mutation analysis is available in MS, but the diagnosis is essentially based on clinical evaluation. *FBN2* mutation confirms Beals syndrome. Serum amino acids demonstrating elevated methionine and homocysteine and low cysteine is the recommended screening test for homocystinuria, but false negatives do arise.

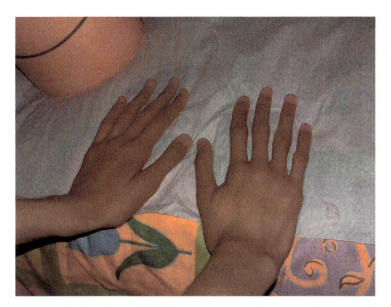

Figure 9.5 Arachnodactyly is clearly present in this patient, referred as a case of Marfan syndrome, but whose other clinical findings did not substantiate the diagnosis.

9.6 Camptodactyly

Recognizing the Sign One or more fingers is held in a flexed position at one or more joints. The fifth finger is most commonly affected and the proximal interphalangeal joint is the most likely joint to be involved.

Establishing a Differential Diagnosis Establish whether the joint abnormalities are local or generalized by evaluating joint function generally. In so doing, take the opportunity to assess tone, power, and reflexes. Most forms of camptodactyly involving multiple joints arise from **fetal akinesia**, the major causes of which are central nervous system (CNS) abnormality, anterior horn cell abnormality, and muscle disease. Pinpointing a specific diagnosis is usually a function of detailed radiologic, neuropathologic, and genetic studies. A history of mild maternal weakness may be the sole clue to the underlying cause of severe multiple joint camptodactyly in an infant who has **maternal myasthenia syndrome**, the mother being, in most instances, previously undiagnosed with myasthenia gravis. There are clinically identifiable syndromes that present with camptodactyly. A small mouth, particularly if associated with an H-shaped ridge of skin over the chin and deep-set eyes, should prompt the diagnosis of **Freeman-Sheldon syndrome** in a camptodactylic neonate. Likewise, ear malformations, typically involving a loss of definition of the upper helical region, and additional folds of tissue conferring a "crumpled" appearance suggest **Beals congenital contractural arachnodactyly (CCA) syndrome** as the diagnosis. The fingers are notably long and large joint contractures, especially of the knees and elbows, are to be anticipated. In the presence of a shawl scrotum, camptodactyly may be explained by **Aarskog syndrome**—look for the characteristic hypertelorism, X-linked history, and periumbilical depression (Figures 2.1A, 8.1A and 9.7B). Micrognathia and/or cleft palate in a neonate with camptodactyly probably signifies the diagnosis of **Catel-Manzke syndrome**. Cardiac evaluation is indicated. The presence of ptosis, orofacial weakness, and clinical impression of a small mouth in a patient who has a history of camptodactyly should prompt evaluation for myotonia. All are well-described features of **Schwartz-Jampel syndrome**, an easily overlooked cause of camptodactyly.

Investigations to Consider Neuroradiology, immunohistochemistry, and molecular studies of muscle disease comprise the mainstay of investigation in undiagnosed camptodactyly presentations. Antibodies specific to the fetal acetylcholine receptor should be undertaken in the mother of a baby with multiple joint contractures. *FBN2* mutation will confirm a clinical diagnosis of CCA. Hand radiology in Catel-Manzke will establish the presence of the hallmark feature, an accessory bone between the proximal phalanges of fingers 2 and 3. Electromyography (EMG) confirms myotonia in Schwartz-Jampel cases. Skeletal radiology in Schwartz-Jampel patients shows platyspondyly with generalized chondrodysplasia.

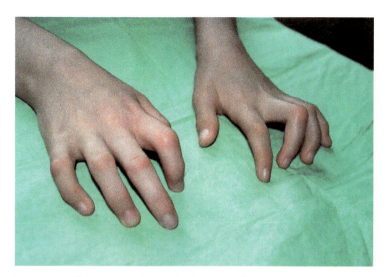

Figure 9.6A Bilateral camptodactyly is demonstrated.

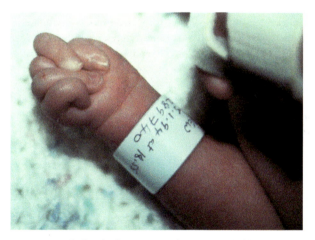

Figure 9.6B The hand of a patient with Freeman-Sheldon syndrome is shown. See also Figure 5.1 for the typical facial appearance and another example of associated camptodactyly.

9.7 Brachydactyly

Recognizing the Sign One or more fingers are short. Generally, the shortening is phalangeal and there may be associated clinodactyly, but the term also covers metacarpal shortening both in combination with phalangeal involvement and in isolation thereof.

Establishing a Differential Diagnosis Both family and pregnancy histories are important. There are several autosomal dominant patterns of brachydactyly, some associated with generalized short stature, which may come to light through family history and examination and explain the clinical features in the patient without recourse to investigation. **Teratogens** tend to cause a brachydactyly of the distal phalanges, important and common culprits being alcohol and phenytoin. Alcohol may be denied, so do assess for accessory palmar creases, additional nipples, short palpebral fissures, thin upper lip, and smooth philtrum, which may lend support to this difficult diagnosis. These causes excluded, think about specific syndromic considerations as follows. If the brachydactyly only involves the thumb, evaluate the birth weight and face for **de Lange syndrome**, in which short first metacarpal is characteristic (Figure 9.13B). Look especially for synophrys, generalized hirsutism and a thin upper lip. Micropenis and/or cleft lip are suggestive of **Robinow syndrome**— evaluate the umbilicus to see if it is displaced toward the sternum and look at the face for hypertelorism. Broad thumbs are frequent, due to duplication of the terminal phalanx. Hypertelorism and brachydactyly but with normal-sized penis should prompt the thought of **Aarskog syndrome**. Specifically, look for the periumbilical depression so typical of this condition and the shawl configuration of the scrotum. Get the patient to close the fist and look for the short fourth metacarpal by observing the knuckle-knuckle-dimple-knuckle sign (the ring finger has a depression over the joint secondary to the shortness of the fourth metacarpal). This sign is the hallmark of familial **brachydactyly type E**, in which development is normal. However, the same sign is often demonstrated in cases of **Albright's hereditary osteodystrophy** (AHO), in which developmental delay, generalized obesity, and signs of hypothyroidism should be sought. Palpate the skin lightly, looking for areas of subcutaneous calcification. Stature is generally short and metatarsal shortening, most commonly of the fourth and fifth metatarsals should also be sought.

Investigations to Consider Hand x-rays may show terminal phalangeal duplication of the thumbs in Robinow cases. *FGD1* gene mutation analysis may confirm a clinical diagnosis of Aarskog syndrome as may *ROR2* analysis in Robinow syndrome. Chromosome 2q37 studies are important in AHO as deletion of this region mimics AHO, true AHO cases having variable hypocalcemia, raised parathyroid hormone levels, and *GNAS1* mutation.

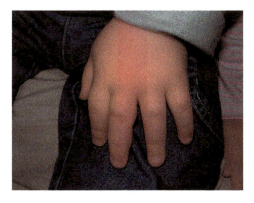

Figure 9.7A Generalized brachydactyly is shown, the noteworthy clinical feature being short nails.

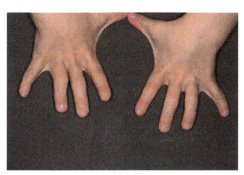

Figure 9.7B By contrast with Figure 9.7A, brachydactyly is associated with partial skin syndactyly, clinodactyly, hyperextension of the metacarpophalangeal (MCP) joints (see how prominent the tendons are over the MCP joints), and flexion of the fourth proximal interphalangeal joint bilaterally. This patient has classical hand features of Aarskog syndrome. See also Figures 2.1A, 8.1A, and 8.7

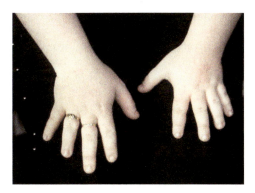

Figure 9.7C The generalized brachydactyly associated with familial brachydactyly type E is demonstrated in this patient.

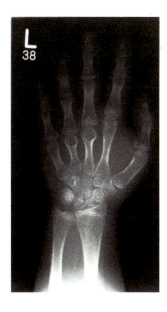

Figure 9.7D The radiograph of the hand from Figure 9.7C confirms the particular shortening of the fourth metacarpal.

9.8 Tapering Fingers

Recognizing the Sign All fingers taper naturally in a proximodistal direction but this ill-defined clinical sign refers to a progressive narrowing of finger breadth, which is noteworthy for the degree of narrowing.

Establishing a Differential Diagnosis Of itself, this sign represents a minor malformation and may be of no clinical significance. Like all minor malformations, the value of the observation is to heighten awareness for other signs that signify an underlying diagnosis. Tapering fingers are well described in association with obesity but are especially characteristic of **Cohen syndrome**. This autosomal recessive condition of truncal obesity and developmental delay has characteristic facial features of a short philtrum, conferring an open-mouthed presentation, prominent central incisors, and a thick head of hair (Figure 2.8). Early-onset myopia and progressive pigmentary retinopathy are valuable supportive signs, without which the diagnosis should be infrequently reached. Unless there is an older affected sibling, this is not a diagnosis for the neonatal period and is more easily made in the 3-year-old and upward age range, at which stage the tapering fingers and truncal obesity are more readily recognizable. Tapering fingers in the neonatal period are uncommon, but if associated with arachnodactyly should result in evaluation for the neonatal presentation of **Marfan syndrome** (MS). Cardiac complications are usually severe and of early onset with aortic root dilatation and valvular dysfunction. Emphysema is a particular complication of this form of MS and assists the diagnosis if identified. Extreme hypotonia in the neonatal period with tapering fingers is the combination of features that facilitates the early diagnosis of **Ehlers-Danlos syndrome (EDS) type VIA** before the characteristic kyphoscoliotic signs appear and make diagnosis easier. The unusual pattern of "criss-cross" lines on the palms and soles is a very valuable, indeed virtually pathognomic, sign (Figure 9.18C). An impression of tapering fingers is common in obese older children, usually with developmental delay, and **chromosomal mosaicism** should be investigated in such a context. Look for linear hypopigmentation, clinically and by ultraviolet light examination.

Investigations to Consider Unexplained neutropenia is a common finding in Cohen syndrome and a valuable aid to diagnosis if present. Retinal examination is indicated for the characteristic pigmentary retinopathy if Cohen syndrome is suspected. Mutation analysis of the *COH1* locus on chromosome 8 will establish the diagnosis, but there may be other unidentified genes. Bone age may be advanced in neonatal EDS VI. Urinary pyridinoline analysis is a very effective test, obviating the need for lysyl hydroxylase assay on fibroblasts. Fibroblast culture is usually necessary to secure a diagnosis of chromosomal mosaicism. Neonatal MS is confirmed by *FBN1* mutation, usually in exons 24–32.

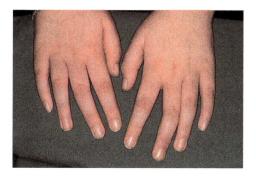

Figure 9.8A A classic example of tapering fingers is shown in this 10-year-old girl with Cohen syndrome.

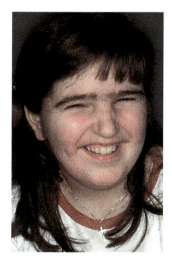

Figure 9.8B Note the thick hair, the manner in which the upper lip retracts on smiling, and the large central upper incisors in the face of the same patient (see also Figure 2.8).

9.9 Puffy Fingers

Recognizing the Sign A purely subjective impression, the fingers appear swollen. Though a rare sign, due to its diagnostic significance its identification can be extremely valuable.

Establishing a Differential Diagnosis The exclusivity of a particular clinical sign to one particular syndrome is unusual, but applies in this instance. Puffy fingers are virtually pathognomonic of **Coffin-Lowry syndrome**. This is an X-linked mental retardation syndrome. Intellectual development is usually severely impaired and early hypotonia and motor milestone delay are typical. The facial appearance, difficult to recognize in the neonatal period, coarsens with time, with hypertelorism and thickened, everted, lips being the most consistent features. There is frequently an associated pectus excavatum. As also occurs in Williams syndrome, there is a propensity to rectal prolapse. The fingers are puffy in appearance and a telling and useful additional sign is the presence of an accessory transverse hypothenar crease on the hand. It should be noted that the fingers are entirely pain free and normally functioning. The family history may offer substance for the diagnosis with other affected males, consistent with X-linked inheritance being identified. Older patients frequently show severe kyphoscoliosis. Clinical examination of females in a pedigree is also warranted, the puffy fingers often being present in obligate carriers. Indeed, the author has seen the diagnosis made in a floppy male neonate by the astute glance that the clinician gave at the carrier mother's hands.

Puffy fingers are also seen in **infantile systemic hyalinosis**, an autosomal recessive condition, but in contrast to Coffin-Lowry syndrome, the fingers in this condition are swollen and painful. There is usually hyperpigmentation over the joints and dermatologic evidence of inflammation, particularly periauricular, perioral, and perianal, is another diagnostically useful distinction.

Investigations to Consider Coffin-Lowry syndrome is a clinical diagnosis. The main sources of diagnostic error are confusion with Williams syndrome, in which the fingers are not swollen but the lip prominence can mislead the inexperienced. Similar scope for confusion arises from the facial resemblance between Coffin-Lowry syndrome and α-thalassemia mental retardation, X-linked (ATRX) syndrome. Staining a blood smear with 1% brilliant cresyl blue in search of hemoglobin H inclusion bodies is a useful screen to exclude the latter. Molecular confirmation of Coffin-Lowry cases is available by *RSK2* mutation analysis.

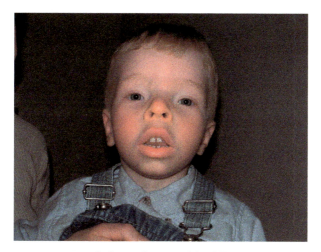

Figure 9.9A Note the hypertelorism and lip fullness in the face of the affected boy with Coffin-Lowry syndrome.

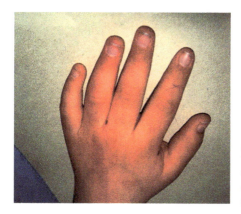

Figure 9.9B The digits are broad and look swollen in this hand of a typical female carrier of Coffin-Lowry syndrome.

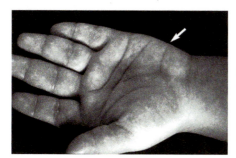

Figure 9.9C The hypothenar crease is shown in a Coffin-Lowry affected boy, but it is worth also observing the generalized puffiness of the fingers. (Courtesy of Professor Ian Young.)

9.10 Overlapping Fingers

Recognizing the Sign This sign is hardly open to misinterpretation, though some overlap with camptodactyly is inevitable. However, camptodactyly is not invariably associated with overlapping position of the fingers, and the reverse also holds true.

Establishing a Differential Diagnosis Overlapping fingers, typically of the index finger over the middle finger and of the fifth finger over the ring finger, is characteristic of **Edwards syndrome** (trisomy 18). Generally, the hands are clenched, the thumb often adducted across the palm. Close inspection frequently shows absence of the distal creases of the fifth fingers. Viewed in profile, the skull is dolichocephalic, with a prominent occiput and low-set ears, usually malformed in appearance. Cardiac examination will establish congenital heart lesions in more than 80% of cases. Much less commonly, overlapping is observed in **Patau syndrome** (trisomy 13), in which condition postaxial polydactyly of the fingers is the more typical finding, sometimes indeed with associated overlapping. The hands of **Pena-Shokeir syndrome** can exactly resemble the hands of trisomy 18 syndrome—this is a condition of multiple joint contractures, paucity of facial movement, and pulmonary hypoplasia, often fatal. Being autosomal recessive, its recognition and clear distinction from trisomy 18, a sporadically occurring condition, is important. Chromosomal disorders aside, overlapping fingers are seen in **Beals congenital contractural arachnodactyly (CCA) syndrome**, in which cases the crumpled appearance of the upper helix of the ear and the joint contractures, especially of the knees, will render the condition readily diagnosable. In a similar vein, **maternal myasthenia syndrome**, already considered under camptodactyly (section 9.6), can present in an infant with fingers whose gross appearance is of overlapping position, but the superficial interpretation of this sign will be modified by examination of joint creases, range of movement, and involvement of other joints in the pathologic process, most particularly in the form of talipes, hip flexion, and knee extension. Multiple joint contractures, particularly if there is ulnar deviation of the hand, the fingers possibly overlapping, is a typical presentation of **Freeman-Sheldon syndrome**, an easily made diagnosis from the facial inspection, the mouth being small and pursed, often with a hallmark H-shaped knuckle of skin over the chin (Figures 5.1 and 9.6). The author has twice made the diagnosis of **Smith-Lemli-Opitz (S-L-O) syndrome** by noting an overlapping index finger in an otherwise nondysmorphic child and investigating biochemically.

Investigations to Consider Basic karyotype is needed for chromosomal trisomies. *FBN2* mutation analysis is indicated for CCA. Antifetal-type acetylcholine receptor antibodies are warranted in suspected maternal myasthenia syndrome. Low serum cholesterol and elevated 7-dehydrocholesterol typify S-L-O.

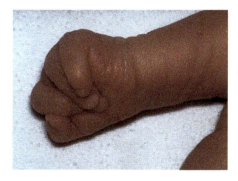

Figure 9.10A The hands of a case of Edwards trisomy 18 syndrome are shown. Note the position of the index finger overlapping the middle finger, the flexed thumb, and the fifth finger overlapping the fourth. The nails are also hypoplastic. (Courtesy of Professor Ian Young.)

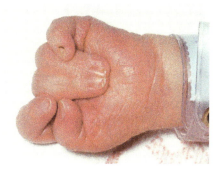

Figure 9.10B The hands of a different case of Edwards syndrome, demonstrating overlapping fingers, small nails, and syndactyly. (Courtesy of Professor Ian Young.)

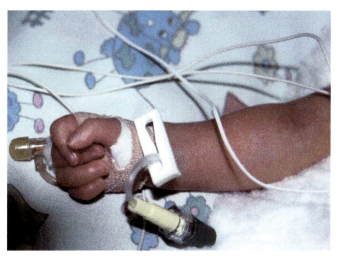

Figure 9.10C The hands of a child with Smith-Lemli-Opitz syndrome are demonstrated showing the occasional finding in that condition of the index finger overlapping the middle finger.

9.11 Ectrodactyly

Recognizing the Sign There is absence of central digits, perhaps extending to involvement of the metacarpals, and often demonstrating syndactyly, camptodactyly, or clinodactyly of the remaining digits.

Establishing a Differential Diagnosis Start with a detailed family history. The condition of **ectrodactyly, ectodermal dysplasia, and clefting (EEC) syndrome** is an autosomal dominant condition of wide clinical variability, and many aspects such as dry skin, palmar hyperkeratosis, small brittle nails, sparse hair, and hypodontia need to be evaluated in attempting to identify a history of this disorder. Reports of tear duct anomalies in family members are a valuable diagnostic clue. In examining the patient, evaluate all four limbs. The extent of limb involvement need not be equally severe in all limbs for this diagnosis to be reached. Cleft lip is common in affected individuals. Blue irides and photophobia are useful supportive clues to observe. It is valuable to examine the hands and feet of parents, whose digits may be normal but have abnormal skin grooves of the palms of feet, betraying mutation carrier status. The allelic condition of **limb mammary syndrome** (LMS) differs in that the ectrodactyly is associated with hypoplasia of the nipples and mammary glands but there is no clefting or signs of ectodermal dysplasia and lacrimal duct anomalies are much less common. Genetically distinct syndromes of **split hand and foot malformations** (SHFMs) not involving ectodermal signs are usually identifiable from the autosomal dominant family history. Cup-shaped ears are often observed in this situation as is limb shortening, especially of the tibia and/or ulna. Clinical overlap in terms of limb shortening or asymmetry between the limbs and the appearance of an ectrodactyly-like malformation of the hand occurs between SHFM and **femur-fibula-ulnar (FFU) syndrome**. The hand appearance in FFU syndrome usually reflects absence of the digits on the ulnar side of the hand. Likewise, an ectrodactyly-like hand is an occasional presentation in **de Lange syndrome**, but the low birth weight, microbrachycephaly, general hirsutism, and characteristic synophrys should facilitate differentiation from other causes of ectrodactyly. Seen in association with holoprosencephaly or anencephaly, ectrodactyly is signaling the diagnosis of **XK aprosencephaly syndrome,** an important condition to recognize since there is evidence that some such families represent autosomal recessive inheritance.

Investigations to Consider Mutation analysis of *P63* on chromosome 3q27 confirms the diagnosis of EEC syndrome and LMS.

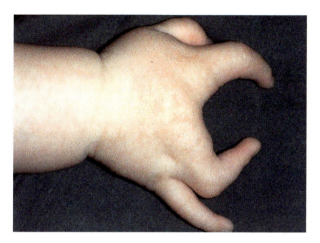

Figure 9.11 A typical "lobster-claw" malformation of EEC syndrome showing, in addition to the ectrodactyly, camptodactyly of the digits on either side of the cleft.

9.12 Broad Thumbs

Recognizing the Sign There is no definition as such, but in addition to looking broad with respect to the other digits, the thumb may present a flattened appearance, perhaps with abnormal angulation of the terminal phalanx.

Establishing a Differential Diagnosis Though not exclusive of other diagnoses, broad thumbs are quintessentially associated with two syndromes of which they represent the hallmark feature. These are Rubinstein-Taybi syndrome and Pfeiffer syndrome. In **Rubinstein-Taybi syndrome,** there is often radial angulation of the terminal phalanx of the thumbs. Examine the feet for associated hallucal broadening. Microcephaly is usual, the forehead being prominent and the palpebral fissures downslanting. The nose is absolutely characteristic, the nasal bridge being wide and the columella extending below the ala nasi (Figure 2.5B). Generally recognizable in the newborn period, these features become more pronounced with age. A small number of cases have been diagnosed molecularly in whom the facial characteristics prompted the diagnosis but the thumbs were normal. These represent an exception in what remains a clinical diagnosis. **Pfeiffer syndrome** comprises the association of craniosynostosis and broad thumbs. Hallucal broadness is usual and some soft tissue syndactyly of the hands and feet common. The craniosynostosis is generally a brachycephaly due to underlying coronal suture fusion, but more extensive malformation is possible, including the severe clover-leaf skull malformation. Being autosomal dominant, careful assessment of the parents and family may identify others affected. Complete syndactyly giving the "mitten" appearance in association with broad thumbs is diagnostic of **Apert syndrome**, another of the craniosynostosis group of disorders, but which represents a sporadically occurring new dominant mutation. Both Pfeiffer and Apert syndromes may have associated joint fusions, especially of the elbow and radioulnar joints. In association with short stature, broad thumbs are often the clue to the diagnosis of **Robinow syndrome**. The genitalia should be examined, often being small, though sex assignment is usually clear. A very useful sign in the neonatal period is gum hypertrophy. Finally, the pitfall of interpreting this clinical sign in isolation of a family history and relevant clinical observation is exemplified by three cases in the author's experience whose real diagnosis of autosomal dominant **brachydactyly type D** was misattributed to Rubinstein-Taybi syndrome and the family wrongly advised of the inevitability of severe mental retardation.

Investigations to Consider Skull x-ray is warranted if craniosynostosis is a concern. Sleep studies should be conducted for sleep apnea in craniosynostosis syndromes. Hand radiology in Robinow syndrome may show bifid terminal phalanges of the thumb and index finger. *FGFR1/2/3* mutation analysis is indicated in craniosynostosis depending on the exact phenotype suspected.

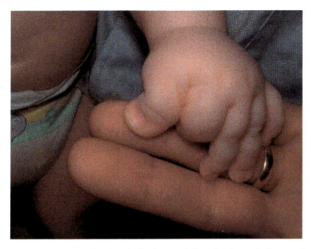

Figure 9.12A Broad and radially deviated thumb of a typical case of Rubinstein-Taybi syndrome is demonstrated.

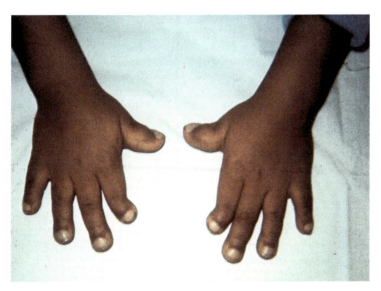

Figure 9.12B The short, broad, radially deviated thumbs bilaterally are shown in a case of Pfeiffer syndrome. Note also the brachydactyly of the index fingers.

9.13 Small and Hypoplastic Thumbs

Recognizing the Sign There is quite a wide range of clinical presentations, from the clinically small but functionally normal thumb to the functionally useless pedunculated digit. If in doubt, assess the length of the thumb by seeing how far it reaches along the radial border of the hand. A thumb that does not reach the metacarpophalangeal (MCP) joint of the index finger is short. Thenar eminence hypoplasia is usual with this sign.

Establishing a Differential Diagnosis A prenatal history of polyhydramnios should be sought, as unilateral thumb hypoplasia may be the sole finding on external clinical examination in **VATER association** (*v*ertebrae, imperforate *a*nus, *t*racheo*e*sophageal fistula, *r*adial +/– renal anomalies). Vertebral anomalies, anal stenosis/malposition, and cardiac malformations should be the subjects of particular examination, especially if a tracheoesophageal fistula/atresia is established. Symmetrically hypoplastic but clinically identifiable thumbs associated with forearm shortening, the consequence of radial aplasia, are typical of **thrombocytopenia-aplastic radii (TAR) syndrome**. Neonatally symptomatic thrombocytopenia should be anticipated in most cases of this autosomal recessive condition. Examine the lower limbs for corroborative signs such as limb asymmetry, limb bowing, or hip dislocation. Cow's milk intolerance is a surprising and unexplained feature of many TAR patients. It is advisable to examine the heart in patients with thumb hypoplasia. A murmur, particularly an atrial septal defect (ASD), should raise diagnostic consideration of **Holt-Oram syndrome** (HOS). Bilateral hand involvement is usual in this autosomal dominant condition, but the hand malformations are quite variable and can be asymmetric. Associated syndactyly, phocomelia, and thumb triphalangy are well within the spectrum of the condition and should be sought in other family members, unsuspecting of their risk of possible cardiac lesions. In a healthy child with thumb hypoplasia, assess for short stature and café-au-lait patches or abnormal skin pigmentation. These cutaneous signs are valuable pointers toward the autosomal recessive condition of **Fanconi pancytopenia syndrome**, the pancytopenia and associated leukemia rarely presenting before the age of 8 or 9 years, but the condition can be anticipated from the other features. Being autosomal recessive, early recognition has clinical implications for predictive testing in siblings. In **de Lange syndrome**, the thumbs often appear short, due to the short first metacarpal bone, which is a hallmark of the condition.

Investigations to Consider Vertebral radiology and echocardiography are indicated in suspected VATER association, and platelet count in TAR syndrome. Echocardiogram and ECG are used to confirm HOS. Chromosome breakage studies following diepoxybutane (DEB) exposure confirms Fanconi syndrome.

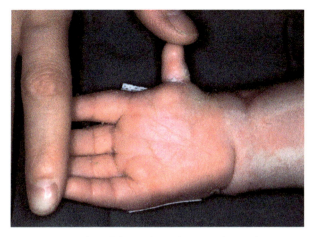

Figure 9.13A Unilateral thumb hypoplasia in a boy with VATER association. Note the absence of any thenar prominence.

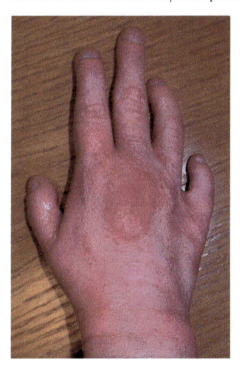

Figure 9.13B The short thumb, consequent on shortening of the first metacarpal bone, is shown in a typical example of Cornelia de Lange syndrome. Note that the other fingers are of normal length. The thumb does not extend to the MCP joint of the index finger, which is a good indicator of shortening. (Courtesy of Professor R.C. Hennekam.)

9.14 Long and Triphalangeal Thumbs

Recognizing the Sign Thumb length is assessed by holding the thumb in parallel with the hand and establishing how far along the index finger the thumb extends. Long thumbs extend to or beyond the proximal interphalangeal (PIP) joint of the index finger. Reduced thenar musculature is usual.

Establishing a Differential Diagnosis Digitized thumbs, possessed of a triphalangeal constitution, are particularly associated with deafness, congenital anemia, and structural heart defects. There is generally bilateral hand involvement, though the nature of thumb malformation can be variable, perhaps being digitized on the one side and duplicated or hypoplastic on the other. Examine the external ears—simple or cup-shaped ears with thumb malformations/digitization suggest a diagnosis of **lacrimo-auriculo-dento-digital (LADD) syndrome**. Delayed eruption of teeth, absent teeth, and failure to produce tears on crying are valuable corroborative evidence of this diagnosis, in which deafness is to be anticipated. While cup-shaped ears are more reminiscent of LADD syndrome, the presence of preauricular tags or pits in the context of thumb triphalangy is more likely to represent **Townes-Brocks syndrome** (T-BS). Anal malformations, including stenosis, anterior placement, and fistulae, are a central element of the diagnosis in patients with this autosomal dominant condition. While an individual case may personally show no anal features, the family history may offer the evidence needed to secure the diagnosis. Examination of the cranial nerves is important in cases of thumb digitization, unilateral sixth nerve palsy with contralateral enophthalmos (Duane phenomenon) being the best clinical sign to the diagnosis of **Okihiro syndrome**. This may present in the neonate as a strabismus. Deafness and renal malformations should be sought. Thumb elongation can be the presenting feature of **Blackfan-Diamond syndrome**, in which a congenital hypoplastic anemia occurs. While most individuals with this condition have normal hands, the thumb abnormality, if present, can be the prompt to diagnosis. In relation to congenital heart disease, the variable nature of hand abnormalities in **Holt-Oram syndrome** (HOS) does extend to long/digitized thumbs, so careful cardiac evaluation and family history are needed before this possible diagnosis can be discounted.

Investigations to Consider Audiologic assessment is needed, as is renal ultrasound, especially if T-BS is suspected. Hematologic indices are warranted. Echocardiogram and ECG are indicated for HOS. Mutation analysis of *SALL1* for T-BS and *SALL4* for Okihiro syndrome should be considered.

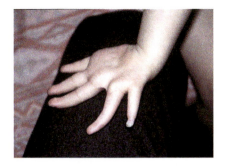

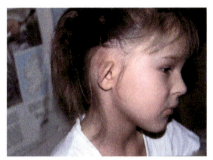

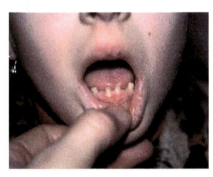

Figure 9.14A–C The digitized thumb, cup-shaped ear, and hypodontia shown here were all seen in a patient with LADD syndrome. Note the abnormal configuration of the hand and the abnormal thumbnail.

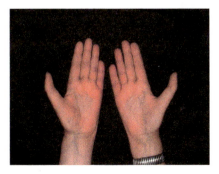

Figure 9.14D A more typical example of thumb triphalangy is shown from an adult deaf patient with Townes-Brocks syndrome. Note the abnormal angulation of the thumbs, the flattened thenar eminence, and the elongated proximal phalanx, which was confirmed radiologically as two fused phalanges.

9.15 Trident Hand

Recognizing the Sign The description refers to a triangular configuration of the hand, caused by short broad fingers. The net effect of phalangeal shortening is a splaying of the fingers, the index and ring fingers pointing away from the middle finger. This confers a three-pronged, "trident," appearance.

Establishing a Differential Diagnosis In contrast to most signs featured between these covers, the trident hand sign is almost exclusive to **achondroplasia**. This is the most common form of chondrodysplasia and usually identifiable at birth. Birth length can extend into the normal range, an important observation that limits the diagnostic usefulness of ultrasonic screening for the condition in pregnancy. Rhizomelic shortening of the humeri is usually noticeable at birth (Figure 11.2A). Coupled with the typically enlarged occipitofrontal circumference, prominent forehead, depressed nasal bridge, and trident hand, skeletal investigations are indicated to secure the diagnosis. In the older child, leg bowing, limitation of elbow extension, and exaggerated lordosis with protuberance of the buttocks all comprise elements of the phenotype. While delay in achieving early motor milestones is usual, normal intellectual outcome is to be anticipated. Foramen magnum compression is an important complication of which to be aware, and sudden death in childhood has been widely reported. Brainstem compression may present as obstructive sleep apnea. The best clinical test for cord compression is to look for clonus and hyperreflexia in the lower limbs. Mental retardation in achondroplasia should result in examination for acanthosis nigricans, seen in **SADDAN syndrome** (severe achondroplasia, developmental delay, acanthosis nigricans). **Thanatophoric dysplasia** also causes a trident hand but the severe compromise of the chest and skeletal system results in an early perinatal death. A cloverleaf skull appearance, due to craniosynostosis, is often present, facilitating the diagnosis ultrasonographically during antenatal life and clinically if the baby is born.

Investigations to Consider Skeletal radiology confirms the diagnosis. The classical radiologic sign of achondroplasia is absence of the normal increase in interpedicular distance from the upper lumbar vertebrae caudally. The pedicles are short, seen on a lateral view, with a narrow vertebral canal. The tubular bones are short and thickened, the fibula often being disproportionately long relative to the tibia. Mutation of *FGFR3* shows a highly specific G1138C, resulting in a Gly380Arg substitution in over 95% of cases, the mutation invariably arising on the paternal chromosome and having a positive association with advanced paternal age. *FGFR3* mutation is also the basis of thanatophoric dysplasia and the classic radiologic sign is bowing of the long bones with "telephone receiver"–shaped femora. SADDAN syndrome represents another form of *FGFR3* mutation, occasioning Lys650Met substitution.

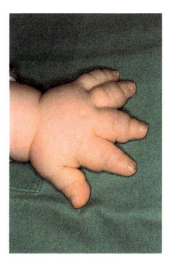

Figure 9.15 The typical appearance of trident hand is demonstrated in a patient who has achondroplasia.

9.16 Fetal Finger Pads

Recognizing the Sign In human embryology fingertip pads arise on the volar surfaces of the fingers but regress in early gestation. The absence of normal regression results in the persistence of fetal finger pads. These are best seen by looking at the fingertips in profile and the well-defined elevation of tissue overlying the terminal phalanges is easily identifiable.

Establishing a Differential Diagnosis The sign is a hallmark feature of two conditions—Kabuki syndrome and Weaver syndrome—but may also be seen as an occasional finding in other pediatric situations. Characteristic facial features facilitate the diagnosis of **Kabuki syndrome** cases—observe the palpebral fissure and note whether it is wide. A good clue is to look for blood vessels in the outer canthus of the eye, where they are not usually seen (Figure 3.14). The eyebrows may be unusual, often showing a hairless gap in the middle. Look for ectropion of the lower eyelid, a most uncommon feature in pediatric populations but very characteristic in this diagnosis. Lip pits, cleft palate, and congenital heart disease should be sought. In the older child, short stature may be the presentation and evidence of developmental delay is to be expected. Obesity is characteristic of the syndrome in the adolescent age range. The author has twice made the diagnosis in unsuspected cases of mentally retarded females with short stature referred for assessment on foot of early breast development. By contrast, the history in **Weaver syndrome** is of abnormally high birth weight, overgrowth, and macrocephaly. A hoarse cry is characteristic and developmental delay usual. The facial features are not specific, but forehead prominence, hypertelorism, and a well-formed philtrum are usual, while the chin tends to be somewhat small. Apart from the finger pads, camptodactyly, broad thumbs, and general fleshiness of the hands are consistent with the diagnosis. This is neither a common nor an easy diagnosis to make and overlaps with cases of **Sotos syndrome**. Persistence of finger pads is also recorded as a finding in several clinically nonspecific chromosomal deletion syndromes, but one in particular, **deletion 22q13** (as distinct from 22q11 deletion), repays specific investigation in children with mild mental retardation but disproportionate delay in speech.

Investigations to Consider Kabuki syndrome is a clinical diagnosis. Advanced bone age should be sought if Weaver syndrome is clinically likely. Mutation analysis of *NSD1*, the Sotos syndrome locus, is positive in some but not all cases of Weaver syndrome. 22q13 deletion requires customized cytogenetic investigation by subtelomere study or, if available, array-based comparative genomic hybridization.

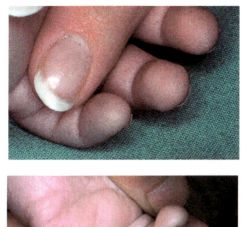

A

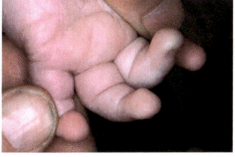

B

Figure 9.16A and B The fetal finger pads are well demonstrated in both cases of Kabuki syndrome shown here. See Figures 3.14 and 3.15 for facial features of Kabuki syndrome.

9.17 Ulnar Ray Defects

Recognizing the Sign There are five digital rays, represented by the meta-carpal bones and the digits. By definition, ulnar ray defects comprise malformations of the ring and/or little finger, which may extend to involvement of the metacarpal bones and, occasionally, the ulna.

Establishing a Differential Diagnosis A positive family history of little finger hypoplasia or absence immediately suggests that the presentation represents the autosomal dominant condition **ulnar-mammary syndrome** (UMS). Anal examination may establish abnormal position or stenosis, both corroborative features of the diagnosis. Look specifically at the nipples and breasts, usually hypoplastic, occasionally absent. Genital hypoplasia should be sought in males. Older patients may have delayed puberty, and the absence of apocrine glands typically results in reduced axillary sweat production. In the presence of symmetric bilateral ulnar ray defects, the main alternative syndromic consideration is of **Miller syndrome**. This rare autosomal recessive condition is typified by malar hypoplasia and lower eyelid ectropion, often with an associated eyelid coloboma. While these facial characteristics are easily confused with Treacher Collins syndrome, indeed the ears also being dysplastic as in that disorder, the absence of the fifth finger, often with some syndactyly of the other digits, is the clinical clue that seals the true diagnosis. Reflecting the clinical presentation of the hands, the fifth toes are usually deficient in Miller cases. Ulnar ray defects are described in **diabetic embryopathy**, for which reason a history of maternal diabetes combined with this clinical finding should spark appropriate investigations for other features of that protean condition. This form of oligodactyly has occasionally been described in **de Lange syndrome**, but proximally placed thumbs (Figure 9.13B) and small hands and fingers are more typical hand findings. Nonetheless, in the context of low birth weight, subsequent growth deficiency, and mental retardation, it is not inappropriate to consider this condition in the presence of ulnar ray defects.

Investigations to Consider Mutation analysis of the *TBX3* locus will confirm UMS if necessary, and endocrine investigations may be required in the event of delayed puberty. Miller syndrome is a clinical diagnosis but should be supplemented by echocardiography and radiology of the vertebral column in view of the occasional reports of nonspecific congenital heart disease and vertebral segmentation defects.

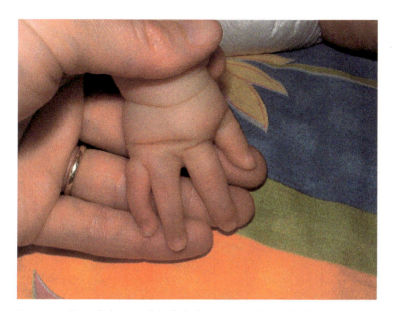

Figure 9.17 Typical absence of the little finger in a patient with ulnar-mammary syndrome. The oligodactyly was bilateral. Note the normal thumb and other digits, absence of syndactyly, and normal joint creases.

9.18 Palmar Crease Patterns of Special Diagnostic Significance

Recognizing the Sign Normal palmar crease patterns accommodate a legion of variation. Typically there are three main creases, a thenar crease, a transverse proximal palmar crease, and a distal palmar crease. No clinical pattern involving the palmar creases is absolutely pathognomic, but particular syndromic significance appertains to a few: (1) deep palmar creases, (2) accessory hypothenar crease, (3) criss-cross patterning, (4) rudimentary palmar crease, and (5) hockey-stick sign.

Establishing a Differential Diagnosis Deep palmar creases, usually with attendant redundancy of the skin, conferring the appearance of an oversized glove is typical of **Costello syndrome**. An early history of poor feeding, high birth weight, and early recognition of developmental delay are useful diagnostic adjuncts. From around the age of 6 years, the typical warty papillomata around the nose and mouth appear and confirm the diagnosis. A clinical overlap with **cardio-facio-cutaneous (CFC) syndrome** exists in that deep creases characterize both disorders and absolute distinction between these entities can be difficult in the first year or two of life. Pulmonary stenosis and hepatomegaly are more likely to signify CFC syndrome. The observation of an accessory hypothenar crease raises the possibility of **Coffin-Lowry syndrome**, an X-linked mental retardation condition with attendant facial features of hypertelorism and prominent, everted lips, becoming more prominent with age (Figure 9.9). Criss-cross patterning of the hands is an unusual appearance often observed in patients with the oculoscoliotic form of **Ehlers-Danlos syndrome type VI**. A blue scleral tinge, prominent eyes that may not close fully during sleep, and evidence of scoliosis should be sought. Rudimentary palmar creases, particularly in the midpalmar region, are sometimes seen in **fetal alcohol syndrome** and can be an important pillar of diagnosis of this clinically elusive condition, but only if supported by other features that frequently attend this condition. Look especially for a featureless philtrum, microcephaly, and short palpebral fissures. A history of neonatal irritability and low birth weight is likely to apply if this is the true diagnosis. Likewise, a hockey-stick sign is also well described in **fetal alcohol syndrome,** referring to the course of the distal palmar crease, pursuing a horizontal course on the ulnar side of the hand and then abruptly angulating to exit between the index and middle fingers.

Investigations to Consider Echocardiography is indicated in Costello syndrome or CFC syndrome for cardiomyopathy or ventricular thickening and pulmonary stenosis in CFC syndrome. Serial examination for neuroblastoma and rhabdomyosarcoma is indicated for Costello cases. Mutation analysis of *RSK2* is needed to confirm Coffin-Lowry syndrome and facilitate carrier detection in females. Urinary pyridinoline cross-links are indicated in EDS type VI.

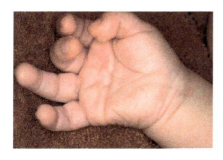

Figure 9.18A The hand of a CFC syndrome case is shown. Note the deep palmar creases.

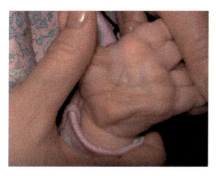

Figure 9.18B Excess, redundant skin in Costello syndrome is shown. Though the palmar creases are not especially deep in this patient, deep creases are also commonly observed in Costello syndrome. See also Figure 2.7B.

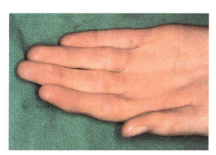

Figure 9.18C This photograph shows the criss-cross pattern so redolent of Ehlers-Danlos syndrome type VI in a patient with that condition. Note the absence of the usual three-crease pattern.

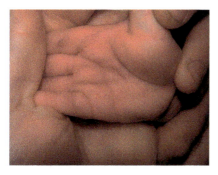

Figure 9.18D Demonstrated is a rudimentary palmar crease between the thenar crease and the distal palmar crease. The usual proximal palmar crease has not formed properly. The distal palmar crease, well established on the ulnar border, represents a hockey-stick configuration. This patient has fetal alcohol syndrome.

Chapter 10 The Feet

10.1 Preaxial Polydactyly

Recognizing the Sign Hallucal reduplication is unlikely to be missed. However, subclinical forms should be suspected in halluces that are clinically broad, the wide toe perhaps representing an underlying duplication of the terminal phalanx, and the clinical sign might be more accurately interpreted as an incomplete duplication.

Establishing a Differential Diagnosis Proximal insertion of an additional hallux that is identifiably distinct from the normally situated hallux is a marker for **diabetic embryopathy,** and such an arrangement of the toes should result in review of the history for maternal diabetes. The family history may yield diagnostically significant information, especially in **Greig syndrome**. The classic description of this autosomal dominant condition, "cephalopolysyndactyly," reflects the main clinical features of macrocephaly, polydactyly, and syndactyly. Typically, the polydactyly is postaxial in the hands and preaxial in the feet, the extra hallux, if fully formed, lying side by side with its companion, perhaps sharing a nail. However, wide variation is well described and seemingly unrelated historical details such as hydrocephalus and absence of the corpus callosum are occasional findings in the syndrome and discounted at the clinician's peril! Familial syndactyly and polydactyly should be targeted in history taking and sought in examining available relatives, as should measurements of occipitofrontal head circumference. Clinically overlapping with Greig syndrome, **acrocallosal syndrome** comprises preaxial polydactyly of both feet, mental retardation, and absence of the corpus callosum. Recognition of this autosomal recessive disorder has important implications for patient and family alike. Examination in cases of preaxial polydactyly is incomplete without looking in the mouth—in particular, evidence of clefting, lingual nodules, or accessory oral frenula raises the possibility of **oro-facio-digital (OFD) syndrome**, of which several genetically distinct subtypes exist. Alternatively, the observation of gum hypertrophy could represent **Robinow syndrome** and further examination for hypertelorism, anteverted nares, short stature, and micropenis give substance to this diagnosis. Plagiocephaly or a family history of craniosynostosis points to a likely diagnosis of **Saethre-Chotzen syndrome**, in which hallucal reduplication is an occasional finding. More typical features to look for are ptosis, incomplete syndactyly of the fingers (Figure 9.3B), and flat forehead.

Investigations to Consider Neuroradiology constitutes an important element of evaluation—absence of the corpus callosum being most likely in acrocallosal syndrome but occasional in Greig cases. Posterior fossa malformations, such as Dandy-Walker abnormality, are described in some of the OFD syndromes. Mutation analysis of the *GLI3* locus establishes the diagnosis of Greig syndrome, while mutation at this locus is reported, albeit rarely, in acrocallosal syndrome. Mutation of *TWIST* confirms Saethre-Chotzen syndrome if in clinical doubt.

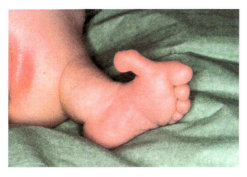

Figure 10.1A Shown is the typical configuration of the preaxial polydactyly of the foot in diabetic embryopathy.

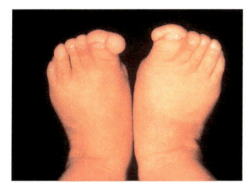

Figure 10.1B Demonstrated are the broad, incompletely reduplicated toes in a case of Greig syndrome.

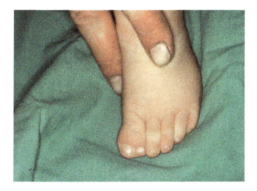

Figure 10.1C This photograph is from a patient with plagiocephaly, which required surgical correction and was due to Saethre-Chotzen syndrome.

10.2 Broad Halluces

Recognizing the Sign The hallux is wider than expected, which may simply be a broad toe or due to underlying phalangeal duplication. The nail, if bifid, is a good clue to incomplete duplication.

Establishing a Differential Diagnosis Examination of the thumbs is no less important. Not only do many of the conditions that cause broad halluces also cause broad thumbs, but also the novice dysmorphologist will often find confidence for diagnostically significant hallucal broadness by looking at the thumbs. **Rubinstein-Taybi syndrome** (R-TS) characteristically shows broad halluces and thumbs, the latter frequently being medially deviated. In the neonatal period, when facial features are less well formed, microcephaly is a valuable adjunctive clinical sign of R-TS. Later, the typical facial features of forehead prominence, broad nasal bridge, and characteristic nose with the nasal columella extending below the level of the ala nasi become evident. In **Pfeiffer syndrome**, the thumbs and halluces are broad, but this autosomal dominant form of craniosynostosis is often recognized within an affected family, whose history may be a valuable aid to correct classification. Look at the skull for evidence of abnormal shape, size of fontanelles, and the configuration of the forehead, which may be flattened or asymmetric. Examine the joints—limitation of elbow movement is an occasional finding in some forms of Pfeiffer syndrome. Broad halluces with plagiocephaly and a positive family history of unusual skull shape or corrective cranial surgery are also typical of a different form of craniosynostosis, **Saethre-Chotzen syndrome** (Figure 10.1C). The clinical distinction between this condition and Pfeiffer syndrome is that the thumbs are normal or possibly even proximally inserted in Saethre-Chotzen cases, but the thumbs of Pfeiffer syndrome are broad. Mild degrees of finger syndactyly are consistent with Saethre-Chotzen syndrome (Figure 9.3B). The broad hallux seen in some instances of **craniofrontonasal dysplasia** (CFND) is invariably accompanied by a longitudinal ridge of the nail, which on cutting, splits neatly at the point of the ridge. Hypertelorism, prominent widow's peak, and a bifid nasal tip are the cardinal facial signs that will identify this condition (Figure 1.7A).

Investigations to Consider R-TS is a clinical diagnosis, but 33% have congenital heart disease, so cardiac evaluation is important in a significant minority. Skull radiology for evaluation of suture patency is fundamental to Saethre-Chotzen, Pfeiffer, and CFND syndromes. Mutation of *FGFR1* or *FGFR2* is likely in Pfeiffer, of *TWIST* in Saethre-Chotzen, and of *EFNB1* in CFND. Sleep apnea studies and optic nerve pressure concerns requiring retinal evaluation are much more likely in Pfeiffer cases than in Saethre-Chotzen or CFND syndromes.

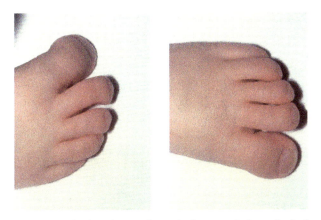

Figure 10.2 The broad toe is shown in the case of a boy who had Pfeiffer syndrome and presented with unusual skull shape and inability to extend the elbow fully at birth.

10.3 Postaxial Polydactyly

Recognizing the Sign An extra digit is manifest on the fibular margin of the foot. It may be unilateral or associated with other digital abnormalities.

Establishing a Differential Diagnosis Examine all four limbs carefully before trying to reach any conclusions. Is there evidence of limb shortening, syndactyly, or brachydactyly? Is the polydactyly mirrored by similar findings in the hand, even of a subtle nature? Once confident that this is an isolated postaxial polydactyly of the feet, whether unilateral or bilateral, commence working toward a diagnosis. From the family history, establish whether this trait is **familial**—the incidence of isolated postaxial polydactyly, of no associated syndromic connotation, is higher in populations of African descent but also observed in Caucasians. Of particular diagnostic concern is the possibility that the extra toe may represent the presenting feature of **Bardet-Biedl syndrome** (B-BS), an autosomal recessive condition. The classic presentation of this syndrome in the older child is a phenotype comprising developmental delay, rod-cone dystrophy resulting in night blindness, hypogenitalism, obesity, and ataxia, sometimes with renal impairment or structural abnormalities of the renal tract predisposing to renal compromise. In full-blown form in the older child, the diagnosis is easily made, but in the neonate, without a family history of an older affected sibling, it is simply not possible to establish the diagnosis, but awareness of this diagnostic possibility and continued observation of the patient are imperative. This need is heightened by the possible high risk of recurrence and the need to establish a diagnosis. **Meckel-Gruber syndrome** if represented by its full clinical constellation of encephalocele/anencephaly, microphthalmia, renal and hepatic cysts, cleft lip and palate, and four-limb postaxial polydactyly is readily identifiable. However, atypical forms arise, usually presenting with renal cysts, polydactyly, and Dandy-Walker malformation of the brain and are less easily recognized, though still representative of autosomal recessive disease and with the attendant risks appertaining in future pregnancies.

Investigations to Consider Serial urea and creatinine levels, as well as urinalysis if abnormal, may be diagnostically important in a possible case of B-BS, apart from the implications of abnormal indices for management. Renal ultrasound may establish evidence for structural changes. Neuroimaging should be considered, especially if head growth, tone, or developmental progress gives cause for concern, and likewise may help secure a diagnosis of B-BS or Meckel/B-BS overlap cases. Mutation analysis is highly unsatisfactory owing to the number of loci and the complexity of interaction between mutations at different loci. Electroretinography (ERG) abnormalities may predate clinical retinal changes indicative of B-BS, not usually seen before age 8 years.

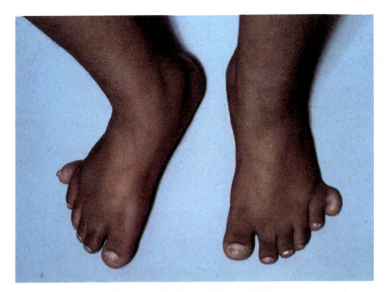

Figure 10.3 The feet of a 7-year-old boy with Bardet-Biedl syndrome are shown. The clinical features of hypogenitalism, suprapubic fat pad, generalized obesity, and developmental delay are apparent by this age.

10.4 Syndactyly of Toes 2/3

Recognizing the Sign The partial or complete fusion of toes 2 and 3 is an easily recognized sign.

Establishing a Differential Diagnosis This is the most common form of **familial syndactyly**, often being associated with partial syndactyly of fingers 3 and 4 either unilaterally or bilaterally. Inheritance is autosomal dominant. Pure syndactyly of toes 2 and 3 without finger involvement also occurs as an autosomal dominant trait, being more common in males. Consequently, this clinical sign has to be interpreted in the context of the family history and appropriate observation of relatives. Though a relatively common clinical sign and not of specific diagnostic significance, its observation can heighten the awareness to additional clinical observations that might otherwise pass unheeded. **Smith-Lemli-Opitz (S-L-O) syndrome** represents a case in point. The facial features of bitemporal narrowing and anteverted nares are easily overlooked on examination, but the combination of hypospadias and 2/3 toe syndactyly will alert the thinking clinician to the possibility of this elusive autosomal recessive cause of mental retardation. Cleft palate should be sought on examination and a particularly valuable clinical clue, if present, is that the index finger may overlap the third finger. Syndactyly of digits 2 and 3 is commonly seen in cases of **Pallister-Hall syndrome**, but the examination of the digits will usually show other features, most typically a polydactyly, perhaps involving both hands and feet. Examination of the anus, which frequently is imperforate, and the mouth for additional frenula offers further evidence for this condition. Similarly, the presence of swallowing difficulties prompting thoughts of tracheoesophageal fistula in a neonate with 2/3 toe syndactyly may denote **Feingold syndrome**. Syndactyly of toes 3 and 4, narrow palpebral fissures, and short index fingers, due to hypoplasia of the middle phalanges, are typical additional clinical findings in this autosomal dominant disorder, where a family history of surgery for tracheoesophageal fistula or duodenal atresia will be strongly suggestive of the diagnosis. Similar clinical findings occur in patients with **deletions of chromosome 13q**. This is, however, a very uncommon condition, and 2/3 toe syndactyly associated with generalized developmental delay can be observed across a wide number of chromosomal deletion or unbalanced rearrangement disorders.

Investigations to Consider Cholesterol is low in S-L-O syndrome, while 7-dehydrocholesterol levels are greatly elevated. Brain imaging is appropriate for Pallister-Hall syndrome to look for the characteristic hypothalamic hamartoblastoma. Dynamic studies of pituitary function may also be indicated. For possible Feingold cases, radiologic and/or endoscopic assessment of the trachea and esophagus are important, as well as excluding a duodenal web. Detailed cytogenetic assessment of chromosome 13q should also be undertaken.

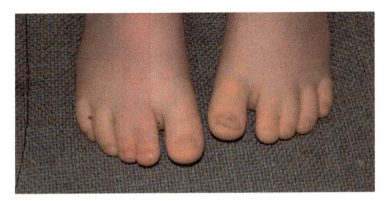

Figure 10.4 Syndactyly of toes 2 and 3, more noteworthy on the right than on the left, is seen in this child. The clinical sign was not pertinent to his developmental delay, as his intellectually normal father also had the same finding.

10.5 Hypoplastic and Missing Toes

Recognizing the Sign Absent toes and hypoplastic toes with or without nail reduction will be easily recognized, but the significance of the sign depends on whether the long bones are normal or otherwise. Short toes may be normal in some forms of skeletal dysplasia. This section addresses short toes unrelated to underlying skeletal abnormalities.

Establishing a Differential Diagnosis Assess all four limbs and identify any other digital abnormalities, in particular absence of fingers, syndactyly, or absent nails. Look for evidence of leg asymmetry, which might be a clue to an **amniotic band disruption** resulting in the digital aplasia. The features will, naturally, vary from case to case, but careful examination may reveal a band-like depression around the lower limb, or specifically around the digit in question, and querying the mother may yield a history of fibrous material bound in a constrictive ring around the base of the missing digit at birth. Some cases overlap with the rare **septooptic dysplasia Pagon type**, in which condition optic nerve hypoplasia is to be expected and pituitary dysfunction an unsurprising accompanying feature. More commonly, the absence of toes heralds a diagnosis of **Adams-Oliver syndrome** (AOS), the observation of aplasia cutis over the scalp being confirmatory (Figure 1.3A). Some syndactyly of the toes or apparent constriction rings are well reported in AOS cases and confer an amniotic band-like configuration on the clinical signs, which may mislead the unwary. AOS is autosomal dominant, for which reason family history and examination may be confirmatory. The range of scalp defects can be very minor, indeed unnoticed by the patient, to severe, requiring surgical intervention. Congenital heart defects have been identified in several cases. Absent fifth toes, usually bilaterally, characterize **Miller syndrome**. The facial features of this condition are reminiscent of Treacher Collins cases, the ears being small and cupped, in addition to a noteworthy malar hypoplasia and eyelid colobomata, but the absence of the fifth fingers and toes clenches the diagnosis. A short hallux, perhaps with an absent nail, may be the harbinger of progressive inappropriate ossification, which characterizes **fibrodysplasia ossificans progressiva**, and may not commence until a few years of age, usually following trauma.

Investigations to Consider If septooptic dysplasia is being considered, neuroradiology to assess the septum pellucidum and midline structures is imperative and dynamic investigation of pituitary integrity ought to be considered. Cardiac evaluation is recommended for cases of AOS, while Miller syndrome patients have a high prevalence of deafness, for which reason formal audiometry is a sensible precaution.

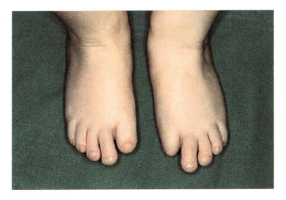

Figure 10.5A The feet of a boy with fibrodysplasia ossificans progressive are shown. The typical bilateral shortening of the halluces is seen, the other toes being normal.

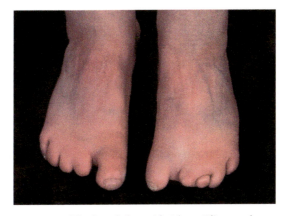

Figure 10.5B The feet of a boy with Adams-Oliver syndrome are shown.

10.6 Longitudinal Plantar Creases

Recognizing the Sign Plantar creases are less well defined than the palmar counterparts, but deep, fissure-like creases in a lengthwise direction along the sole of the foot denote this sign. On questioning the mother, a history is frequently obtained of the deep crevices thus formed as a repository for fluff and the need to actually open the creases out to clean them satisfactorily.

Establishing a Differential Diagnosis Seen as the sole clinically abnormal finding in a neonate, the chances are that the baby has **trisomy 8 mosaicism**. Birth weight, antenatal history, and family history are usually noncontributory in signaling the diagnosis, although the frequent absence of the corpus callosum in the condition may result in abnormality being recognized during antenatal scanning. Occasional cases present clinically with hydrocephalus postnatally. The diagnosis is easily overlooked in the neonatal period, and the pediatric presentation is likely to be of a globally developmentally delayed, nondysmorphic child. In addition to the plantar creases, diagnostically valuable clinical signs that are specifically associated with the condition are dysplastic ears, small patellae, and stiffness of the finger joints, which may progress to contractures with time. Deep creases in the palms should also be sought. **Beare-Stevenson syndrome** is a very rare condition of craniosynostosis, in which the striking malformation of the skull will indicate the underlying diagnosis. Examination of the skin shows acanthosis nigricans and longitudinal wrinkling of the skin, known as cutis gyratum, and this can extend to the feet conferring the appearance of deep plantar creases. Likewise, in **Costello syndrome**, deep plantar creases on the feet can be seen but are not the sole clinical finding, excess skin of the hands and feet, a history of poor feeding in infancy, and the emergence of a coarse countenance toward the end of the first year of life, reminiscent of mucopolysaccharidosis representing sentinel clinical findings. A jowly appearance to the face is typical, as is global developmental delay, and the emergence of nasal papillomata at the age of 5 or 6 years seals the diagnosis (Figure 2.7B).

Investigations to Consider Karyotype is mandatory and, if normal, skin biopsy for karyotype may be necessary to secure confirmation of mosaicism of trisomy 8. Trisomy 8 mosicism becomes more difficult to establish with age, due to the loss of the extra chromosome. Radiology of the knee confirms the absent or small patellae. Mutation analysis of *FGFR2* confirms Beare-Stevenson syndrome, but the diagnosis is essentially clinical. Tumor surveillance is advised in Costello syndrome, the diagnosis of which may be confirmed by mutation analysis at the *HRAS* locus.

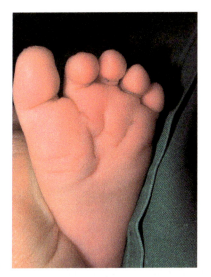

A

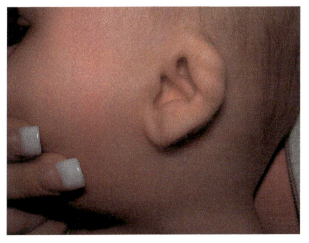

B

Figure 10.6A and B This boy presented to clinic at age 1 year with a history of mild unexplained hydrocephalus and concern that motor milestones were slightly delayed. Indeed, a diagnosis of cerebral palsy had been suggested. Chromosomal study of the blood had been normal in the pediatric clinic. The clinical findings shown, of deep longitudinal plantar creases and dysplastic external ears, prompted skin biopsy and fibroblast karyotype, confirming the diagnosis of mosaic trisomy 8.

10.7 Foot Edema

Recognizing the Sign The characteristic puffiness over the dorsum of the feet is easily recognized. Establish whether there is edema elsewhere, extending up the legs, in the hands, periorbitally, and in the dependent areas. Examine for clinical evidence suggestive of intrauterine hydrops by looking for webbing of the neck and the presence of epicanthic folds.

Establishing a Differential Diagnosis Empirically, the single most likely cause of puffy feet is **Turner syndrome**. Short stature, usually apparent at birth; puffiness over the dorsum of the hands; broad-spaced nipples; and a low posterior hairline, often accompanied by neck webbing, all combine to suggest the diagnosis. Cardiac examination is important because of the high associated prevalence of aortic valve dysplasia and coarctation. **Milroy's disease**, an autosomal dominant form of lymphoedema, almost never presents before the age of 20 years and should be suspected on the basis of the family history of other affected individuals. Likewise, **lymphoedema-distichiasis syndrome** is a condition of postpubertal presentation, in which the autosomal dominant family history and specific evaluation of the upper and lower eyelashes medially for extra hairs establish the diagnosis. Puffy feet in the karyotypically normal neonate may signify **Noonan syndrome,** and additional evidence for this condition may derive from echocardiography, clinical observation of pectus carinatum above and excavatum at the lower end of the sternum (Figure 7.7), as well as evaluation of the parents for history of congenital heart disease and clinical signs of this autosomal dominant condition. **Nephrotic syndrome** may present with puffy feet, which usually transforms into generalized edema fairly quickly, but might be the clinical sign neonatally of the congenital Finnish form, which is autosomal recessive. The neonate with puffy feet needs serial evaluation for development, lest **carbohydrate-deficient glycoprotein (CDG) syndrome** become apparent. In addition to developmental concerns, inversion of the nipples or unusual body fat distribution patterns, such as fat pads over the buttocks, are strong indicators for investigation of this complex of disorders. Any infant with unexplained puffy feet and abnormal tone ought to have an ophthalmic examination looking specifically for optic atrophy, the hallmark of **PEHO syndrome** (*p*rogressive *e*ncephalopathy, *h*ypsarhythmia, *o*ptic atrophy), a rare autosomal recessive disorder.

Investigations to Consider Karyotype is needed to establish 45XO or mosaicism thereof in Turner syndrome. Renal ultrasound is indicated to establish if horseshoe kidney, a frequent Turner associated finding, prevails. Echocardiography should be conducted if Noonan or Turner syndrome is suspected. Coagulation indices are prolonged in Noonan syndrome. Urinalysis is indicated to consider nephrotic syndrome and *NPHS1* mutation analysis to confirm the Finnish form. Isoelectric focusing of transferrin is the best screening measure for CDG syndromes.

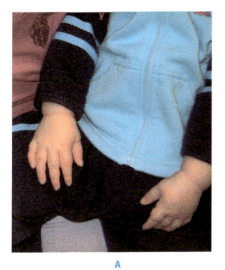
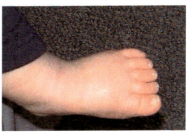

A   B

Figure 10.7A and B Puffy hands and feet from siblings with PEHO syndrome are demonstrated. (Courtesy Dr. Bruce Castle.)

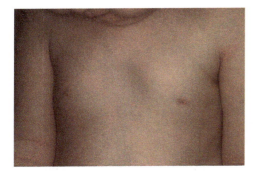

C

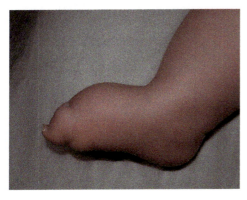

D

Figures 10.7C and D Inverted nipples are shown from a patient with carbohydrate-deficient glycoprotein syndrome type Ia whose initial presentation was with delayed motor milestones and puffy feet (**D**).

10.8 Short Fourth and Fifth Metatarsals

Recognizing the Sign In this clinical sign, the observant clinician notices that the hallux, second and third toes are of relatively normal size but the appearance of the foot is noteworthy for the relative shortness of the fourth and fifth toes. The phalangeal components of these toes are normal and the shortness is established radiologically as a function of short metatarsals.

Establishing a Differential Diagnosis Though not pathognomonic of **Albright hereditary osteodystrophy syndrome**, this sign is especially associated with that disorder and examination should be tailored accordingly. Look for analogous shortening of the metacarpal bones on the ulnar side of the hand. Ask the patient to close the fist and observe whether the metacarpophalangeal joint of the ring finger is foreshortened. In the presence of fourth metacarpal shortening, the fist assumes a characteristic "knuckle-knuckle-dimple-knuckle" configuration. The general body habitus offers clues in that patients are usually short, about two-thirds of cases being below the third percentile for age, and obese. Mental retardation is to be anticipated in the majority of cases. Examination is incomplete without seeking evidence of soft tissue calcification, often concentrated over the scalp and the periarticular regions of the hands and feet. The family history may be of interest, the condition being autosomal dominant, and examination of parental hands and feet illuminating. Confusion with **brachydactyly type E** is the most likely diagnostic pitfall. In this autosomal dominant condition of short stature and normal intelligence, the hands and feet have the exact same appearance as that described in Albright hereditary osteodystrophy cases. However, the absence of mental retardation, obesity, and subcutaneous calcification should facilitate discrimination between these two superficially similar but distinct diagnostic entities. This same clinical sign is observed in the context of mental retardation in a small number of children with **chromosome 2q37 deletion syndrome**.

Investigations to Consider Parathyroid biochemistry is usually distorted in Albright hereditary osteodystrophy. Hypocalcemia and hyperphosphatemia should be sought. Urinary cyclic adenosine monophosphate following stimulation by exogenous parathyroid hormone is usually depressed. Thyroid function should be assessed in view of associated hypothyroidism. Radiology establishes the metacarpal and metatarsal seat of brachydactyly. Mutation analysis of Gs-α subunit establishes the diagnosis if there is clinical or biochemical doubt. Detailed cytogenetics is advised to exclude 2q37 deletion in cases where no mutation is demonstrable or mutation analysis not available.

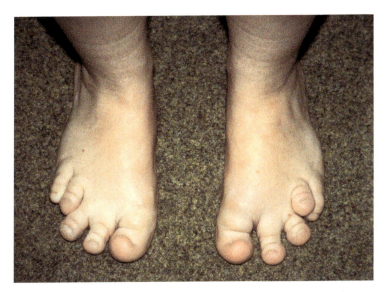

Figure 10.8 The feet of a patient with familial brachydactyly type E are shown.

Chapter 11   The Limbs

11.1 Limb Asymmetry

Recognizing the Sign An anatomically normal limb is noticed to be larger or smaller, longer or shorter than its contralateral counterpart. Having made this observation or perhaps attention having been drawn to it by a mother, the examination seeks to establish whether this is an isolated or more generalized phenomenon. Observe all four limbs for differences. Look at the face for evidence of possible asymmetry. Document any vascular phenomena—hemangiomata, cutis marmorata, or nevi. Measure limb length and girth. A useful question is to establish a discrepancy in shoe size.

Establishing a Differential Diagnosis In the newborn period a hemangioma on the upper lip is a hallmark characteristic of **macrocephaly-cutis marmorata-telangiectasia congenita** (MCTC) **syndrome** (Figure 12.12). Macrocephaly, limb asymmetry, and cutis marmorata, the persistence of a vascular pattern conferring a "marbled" appearance on the skin, are usually present, the latter often becoming more apparent when the baby cries. Developmental delay is usual in patients with this condition. In contrast, **Klippel-Trenaunay-Weber syndrome** (KTW) is characterized by normal development but limb enlargement, which may be of arm or leg only, and is associated with vascular malformations often of a blue or purple color and occasional limb swelling consequent on lymphatic involvement. Serial observation should facilitate differentiation from another condition of normal intelligence and development, **Proteus syndrome**. While many different dermatologic signs may be associated with the latter, the essential hallmarks of the condition are the relentless march of the asymmetry, with progressive overgrowth and resultant disproportion. Macrodactyly of a single finger may emerge. Likewise, in time, the sole of the affected foot may develop a warty, rugose appearance giving the characteristic "moccasin foot." The absence of vascular phenomena and normal intellectual development favors a diagnosis of **isolated hemihyperplasia**. Limb asymmetry is an occasional feature of **neurofibromatosis type 1** (NF1), but the positive family history, clinical signs of axillary and/or groin freckling, and café-au-lait skin patches in the older child will easily facilitate differentiation of this diagnosis from other causes. In the intrauterine growth–retarded baby, limb asymmetry is a good clue to **Silver-Russell syndrome** and relative macrocephaly, poor growth, and the typical triangular-shaped face should be watched for over time.

Investigations to Consider Specialized radiologic approaches to establish associated arteriovenous malformations may be necessary in some cases of KTW syndrome. Wilms tumor screening is recommended for isolated hemihyperplasia cases. NF1 patients need ophthalmic examination in view of the risk of optic glioma, and regular blood pressure recordings are recommended due to the associated risks of phaeochromocytoma and renal artery stenosis.

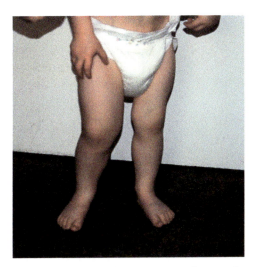

Figure 11.1A Note the discrepancy in size between the enlarged right leg and the normal left leg in this boy aged 18 months. Note the compensatory flexion of the enlarged limb. Absence of skin stigmata narrowed his diagnosis to either nonsyndromic hemihyperplasia or Proteus syndrome, which had yet to declare itself.

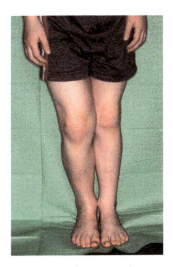

Figure 11.1B The same patient at age 4 years, when a diagnosis of non-syndromic hemihyperplasia had been reached.

11.2 Symmetric Short Limbs

Recognizing the Sign The limbs are short. Note any bowing, perhaps clinically manifest by skin dimpling, which suggests diaphyseal pathology and enlargement of joints, more likely to represent a primary meta-epiphyseal process.

Establishing a Differential Diagnosis Birth length is a useful point of reference by which to assess the changing growth profile. Parental height facilitates the establishment of a "likely height" prediction. Body proportions such as upper-to-lower segment ratios and arm span are valuable in determining whether there is involvement of the axial skeleton in addition to the limbs. Clinically, assess for scoliosis and joint laxity. Observing the limbs, assess by inspection whether the shortening is generalized or more pronounced in one particular region of the limb. Disproportionate rhizomelic shortening, referring to the humeri and femora, is a particular feature of **achondroplasia**, which should be recognizable in the newborn period. In addition to the short limbs, the relative macrocephaly, prominent forehead, and trident configuration of the hands betray the diagnosis on clinical evaluation alone. The observation, during serial review, of atypical features such as acanthosis nigricans should call the original diagnosis into question. The development of acanthosis nigricans in an "achondroplasia" patient indicates **SADDAN (severe achondroplasia, developmental delay, acanthosis nigricans) syndrome**. Clinically and molecularly, the latter condition is closely related to **thanatophoric dysplasia**, associated with very early perinatal death from the narrow chest, but in whom the symmetric short limbs and trident hand closely mimic achondroplasia. Significant chest narrowing also characterizes **Jeune asphyxiating thoracic dystrophy syndrome,** which clinically and radiologically resembles **Ellis–van Creveld (E-vC) syndrome.** Cardiac evaluation will often reveal an atrial septal defect (ASD) in E-vC syndrome. A predominantly mesomelic short-limbed dwarfism, affecting the radius and ulna disproportionately, is typical of patients with **Robinow syndrome,** in whom hypertelorism, anteverted nares, and small genitalia should be sought. Broad or bifid thumbs would likewise support this diagnosis, as would cleft lip. Micrognathia and a persistently palpable fontanelle are the clinical hallmarks of the rare autosomal recessive condition **pycnodysostosis**. The propensity to dental caries, occasional fractures, blue sclerae, and wormian bones on skull x-ray in pycnodysostosis form an obvious pitfall for confusion with osteogenesis imperfecta type I, but the symmetry of the short stature, absence of family history, and skull ossification defect identifiable by persisting patency of the fontanelle should deflect the thinking clinician from this trap.

Investigations to Consider Skeletal radiology and expert interpretation thereof are the gateway to diagnosis. Mutation analysis of *FGFR3* establishes mutations in achondroplasia, SADDAN syndrome, and thanatophoric dysplasia responsible for the different but overlapping patterns of malformation.

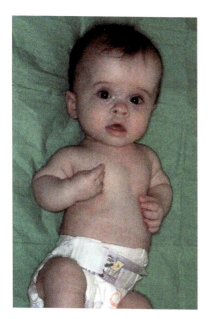

Figure 11.2A A case of achondroplasia is shown. Note the symmetrically short limbs, particularly of the humeri, showing the preferential rhizomelic shortening (proximal bone more severely affected) and the relative macrocephaly. See Figure 9.15 for trident hand.

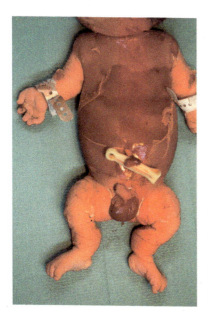

Figure 11.2B A postmortem picture of a case of thanatophoric dysplasia is shown, demonstrating the narrow chest and the abnormal configuration of the lower legs signifying underlying bowing of the bones. (Courtesy of Dr. Peter Kelehan.)

11.3 Limb Reduction Defects

Recognizing the Sign Essentially, this term refers to short, abnormal limbs and incorporates several of the clinical signs already addressed in the chapters dealing with hands and feet. The intention here is to concentrate on conditions predominantly involving the long bones.

Establishing a Differential Diagnosis In addition to a family history, the antenatal history has particular relevance in this situation, with chorionic villous sampling during pregnancy, maternal diabetes, and valproate exposure all being associated with limb reduction defects. Examination of all four limbs is necessary, the intention being to establish whether the abnormality is confined to a single limb or has a more general distribution. **Amniotic bands** will be expected to cause a discernible constriction ring below which the bony and soft tissue growth is distorted by vascular disruption in the single limb affected, all other limbs being normal. The possibility of **Poland anomaly** should be evaluated by examination of the chest for asymmetry, perhaps manifest by the nipples not being in line with one another or the anterior axillary creases being asymmetric between the two sides. In the event of chest asymmetry, examination of the cranial nerves should follow to assess for **Poland-Moebius syndrome**, in which condition mental retardation may occur, in contrast to uncomplicated Poland anomaly. Cranial nerve evaluation is also key to the recognition of **Okihiro syndrome**, an autosomal dominant condition characterized by sixth nerve palsy, deafness, and limb reduction disorders, usually bilateral, but variable. A useful tip is to examine the range of external eye movement in the parents, even if both have normal limbs, as the limb defects can be very subtle and the sixth nerve palsy almost unidentifiable in the baby with the limb reduction defects. Examine the intraoral cavity and assess tongue size—hypoglossia is likely to signify **Hanhardt hypoglossia-hypodactyly syndrome,** and many of these patients also have signs of sixth and seventh cranial nerve damage. Assessment of the scalp is advised, specifically looking for areas of hairlessness signifying cutis aplasia, the hallmark of **Adams-Oliver syndrome,** if there is limb involvement. Cardiac examination may reveal congenital heart disease in Adams-Oliver syndrome, but unless there is identifiable cutis aplasia, is more likely to represent **Holt-Oram syndrome** (HOS), in which autosomal dominant condition the family history of structural heart defects and limb malformations usually prompts the diagnosis.

Investigations to Consider Audiometric assessment is indicated in suspected cases of Okihiro syndrome. Mutation analysis of the *SALL4* gene confirms if the diagnosis is in doubt. HOS cases need electrocardiography (ECG) and echocardiography. Mutation analysis of *TBX5* may be helpful, especially if a new mutation is suspected.

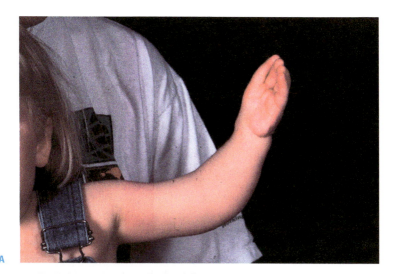

A

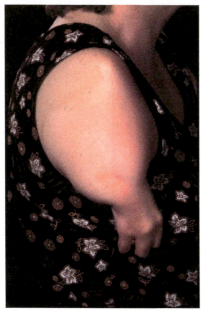

B

Figure 11.3A and B The contrasting limb reduction defects in a daughter and mother with Okihiro syndrome are demonstrated. Lateral rectus palsy on examination of the eye movement was the clue to the diagnosis. See also Figure 7.1B for an instance of amputation-type reduction defect associated with Poland anomaly.

11.4 Localized Lumps on the Limb

Recognizing the Sign In general, genetic causes of localized lumps result in onset of signs after a few years rather than neonatally. Unsurprisingly then, the history is usually of a parent noticing a swelling.

Establishing a Differential Diagnosis The family history may often offer an explanation. Inquiry as to familial tumors or malignancy is advised. Examine for other evidence of previously undocumented lumps. Note the position of lumps, possibly over joints. Establish whether they are mobile, fixed to deeper tissue, or arising from bone. **Neurofibromatosis type 1** is associated with neurofibromata, which present as mobile lumps beneath the skin. Corroborative clinical signs of café-au-lait patches and groin and axillary freckling should be sought. If the diagnosis is established, continuous evaluation throughout childhood for scoliosis and hypertension is usually advised. **Familial angiolipomatosis** is a rare condition in which the lumps are subcutaneous, mimic neurofibromata, and are usually clustered around the joints. The autosomal dominant family history and the absence of other signs of NF1 make this condition very likely. All cases in the author's personal experience have been misdiagnosed as NF1. Lumps that are fixed and clinically of bony origin denote likely **multiple exostoses**. These comprise clinically overlapping autosomal dominant conditions, one of which, on chromosome 11, is associated with craniosynostosis and enlarged parietal foramina, while deletion of chromosome 8q, in addition to the bony lumps, may cause **Langer-Gideon syndrome**. The attendant ala nasi hypoplasia and wispy hair with little temporal hair growth allow clinical recognition of the latter entity. Both forms may be associated with mental retardation. **Cowden syndrome** (CS) is an extremely variable condition often presenting with macrocephaly and developmental delay. A family history of macrocephaly, thyroid malignancy, or fibrocystic breast disease is strongly suggestive. Lumps usually represent hamartomata and are very unpredictable as to clinical presentation and location, some cases being clinically confused with Proteus syndrome. In males, pigmented spots on the glans penis are a very useful clinical sign of this condition. Lumps that are calcified should result in consideration of **Albright's hereditary osteodystrophy** (AHO) as a possible diagnosis and the characteristic brachydactyly of the fourth metacarpal and metatarsal should be sought.

Investigations to Consider Skeletal radiology will confirm multiple exostoses. Parietal foramina on skull x-ray are characteristic of a chromosome 11p deletion. Karyotyping and detailed cytogenetics are appropriate. Deletion 8q should be sought if a Langer-Gideon phenotype prevails. A low threshold for *PTen* mutation analysis is advisable for CS and its clinical variants. Parathyroid and thyroid function tests are indicated for AHO.

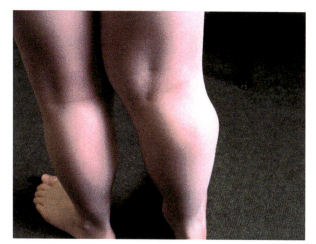

A

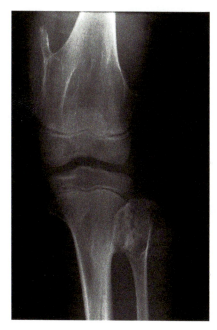

B

Figure 11.4A and B This 8-year-old boy presented acutely due to parental concern about the large swelling on the lateral aspect of his right leg just below the knee. Examination showed several other, previously unnoticed lumps. The family history established that his uncle had had surgical removal of a lump some years previously and histology had shown a cartilage-capped exostosis. Radiology confirmed familial multiple exostoses as the diagnosis. Note the characteristic bony spur on the lower femur, in addition to the large exostosis over the superior tibiofibular joint.

11.5 Arthrogryposis Congenita

Recognizing the Sign Multiple joint contractures are present from birth.

Establishing a Differential Diagnosis Joint contractures may represent a physical manifestation of a primary abnormality in the neuromuscular development of the baby, or may arise secondary to fetal constraint or maternal neuromuscular disease. Hence, family history, with particular reference to talipes or contractures, is important. In particular, maternal history and examination needs to be undertaken. **Myasthenia gravis** in a mother can result in severe arthrogryposis in her offspring. Unsuspected and asymptomatic myasthenia gravis in the mother should be investigated in recurrent cases of fetal arthrogryposis among her offspring. Apart from evaluating the extent of joint limitation, the range of joints affected, and the presence of pterygia (skin webs across affected joints), the clinical examination should also take cognizance of clinical indicators of joint movement in fetal life. Specifically, evaluate the joint creases of the hands and feet, absence of which indicates likely failure to establish movement in early development. Likewise, skin dimples overlying contractures probably indicate failure of normal movement and a primary disease process. General observations with respect to neurologic function may suggest impairment of tone or absence of muscle bulk. **Edwards syndrome**, which frequently presents with clenched hands and overriding fingers as well as limitation of hip movement, should be excluded as the underlying cause. **Amyoplasia congenita** confers a characteristic symmetric malpositioning of joints with talipes equinovarus, flexion of the wrists and fingers, and internal rotation of the shoulders. The presence of dimples and absence of skin creases betrays an absence of normal joint development and movement in utero. A glabellar hemangioma is often present. **Spinal muscular atrophy** (SMA) is easily overlooked as a possible diagnosis, the classic presentation of the disorder being of hypotonia. However, contractures are well described in cases having genetic deletions, so careful attention to feeding history and evaluation for tongue fasciculation may reveal the true diagnosis. **Multiple pterygium syndrome**, an autosomal recessive condition, is usually recognizable at birth because, in addition to multiple large and small joint contractures, pterygia are generally identifiable across the joints. **Beals congenital contractural arachnodactyly syndrome** will be clinically discernible by the characteristic crumpled helix of the ear and arachnodactyly.

Investigations to Consider The anticholinesterase receptor antibody, specific for the fetal receptor is necessary to establish maternal myasthenia syndrome. Karyotype is indicated for Edwards syndrome. Electromyographic study is necessary for SMA and, if in doubt, mutation analysis of the *SMN* locus on chromosome 5 for deletion should be conducted. Mutation analysis of *FBN2* gene confirms Beals syndrome.

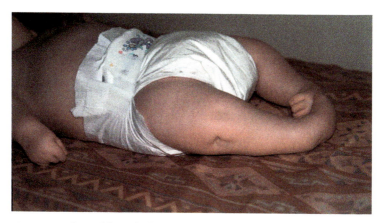

Figure 11.5A Severe bilateral talipes and dimples over the knees are shown in a typical case of amyoplasia congenita.

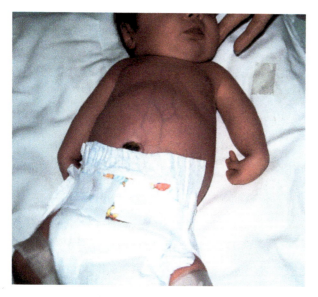

Figure 11.5B Note the wrist flexion and absent elbow joint creases in another patient with the same condition.

11.6 Joint Enlargement

Recognizing the Sign The sign is easily identified, the purpose of examination thereafter being to establish whether the enlargement represents a generalized process involving several joints or whether it is localized to a single joint. If localized, then possible dysmorphic considerations are forestalled by more likely inflammatory causation and evidence of effusion should be sought.

Establishing a Differential Diagnosis The family history is useful; in particular, a family history of conjunctivitis, uveitis, or arthritis should not be discounted. The autosomal dominant condition of **chronic infantile neurologic cutaneous and articular syndrome** (CINCA) presents with an episodic fever and maculopapular rash of neonatal origin, often difficult to diagnose but much more easily recognized if the family history is taken into diagnostic account. Typically painful, swollen joints do not set in until age 3 or 4 years, the knees and ankles being most affected. **Stickler syndrome** is an autosomal dominant condition, and large painless knees in a child with short stature should lead to consideration of this diagnosis. A history of micrognathia, personal or family history of myopia, or retinal detachment and evidence of joint laxity or early-onset osteoarthritis all weigh heavily in favor of this diagnosis. Formal eye evaluation for cataract, vitreous abnormality, and retinal detachment is advised for management as well as diagnostic purposes. In a similar vein, **Kniest syndrome** should be suspected in a child with short stature and large knees. The condition can be suspected neonatally by the relative macrocephaly, symmetrically enlarged knees, and frequent observation of cleft palate. Generalized joint thickening emerging over the first few years of life, often with associated restriction in the range of movement, is characteristic of the joint enlargement that accompanies **mucopolysaccharidosis**, but the typical facial features and usual developmental delay invariably facilitate diagnosis and predate the emergence of this sign. **Multiple exostoses,** discussed in section 11.4, may present with single or multiple periarticular swelling due to the preferential development of exostosis near the epiphyses or the epiphyseal/metaphyseal junction. Finger clubbing associated with symmetric swelling of large joints, particularly the ankles and knees, and excessive palmar sweating is characteristic of **cranio-osteoarthropathy**, an autosomal recessive condition. Cranial suture closure is delayed, with clinical preservation of an open fontanelle until age 2 or 3 years.

Investigations to Consider Radiologic evaluation in Stickler syndrome demonstrates metaphyseal widening, coronal clefts, and platyspondyly in the neonatal period, while a similar finding but with an additional ossification center of the distal end of the middle phalanges typifies Kniest syndrome. Mutations of *COL2A1* cause Kniest, while Stickler syndrome maybe caused by either *COL2A1* or *COL11A1*.

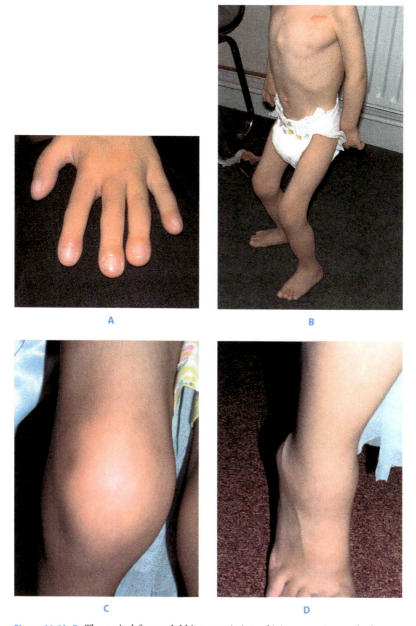

Figure 11.6A–D The typical finger clubbing, restriction of joint extension at the knees, knee enlargement, and ankle swelling of cranio-osteoarthropathy are demonstrated in these illustrations from two different patients with the condition. (C and D courtesy of Dr. Mohnish Suri. Figure reproduced with consent from O'Connell et al. *Clin Dysmorphol* 2004;13:213–219.)

11.7 Generalized Joint Hypermobility

Recognizing the Sign Patients will tend to show you that they are "double-jointed" by demonstrating that they can passively appose the thumb against the flexor aspect of the forearm. Further objective evidence to look for on examination includes passive extension of the fifth metacarpophalangeal joint to greater than 90 degrees, hyperextension of the elbows and knees by greater than 10 degrees, and ability to touch the floor with the palms while standing with the knees extended, by flexing the spine.

Establishing a Differential Diagnosis In view of the major management implications relating to aortic root dilatation, it is critical to establish whether joint hypermobility is indicative of **Marfan syndrome** (MS). Family history may assist, the condition being autosomal dominant. Particular awareness of unexplained deaths in childhood or early adult life is advised, possibly reflecting demise from aortic dissection. Ophthalmic evaluation for myopia and lens dislocation is essential, while clinical signs to observe are pectus; arachnodactyly; an arm span exceeding standing height; high, arched palate; and transverse striae of the skin best sought over the lumbar region. Joint laxity is a feature of **Stickler syndrome** in the pediatric age range, though usually less so in adult life. A history of Pierre-Robin sequence should be sought and clinical evidence of depressed nasal bridge, large knee joints, and a personal and family history of myopia, cataract, or retinal detachment are the central elements of sifting out this diagnosis from other causes of joint laxity. Ligamentous laxity can be familial, and such an observation by history or personal demonstration of signs in a parent is consistent with the **Ehlers-Danlos syndrome** (EDS) complex of disorders. All are genetic, the commoner forms being autosomal dominant. Gorlin sign—the ability to touch the tip of the nose with the tongue—is more common in EDS patients than the general population. Other diagnostically valuable manifestations of EDS are blue sclerae, skin hyperextensibility, easy bruising, scarring disproportionate to the degree of trauma, joint dislocation, surgery for inguinal hernia, and a history of delayed early motor milestones but with normal intelligence. Ophthalmic examination may indicate keratoglobus in type VI, the cornea being prone to rupture on minor trauma. Kyphoscoliosis is a clinical finding among most types, but a signature of type VI and the criss-cross pattern of hand skin in this particular variant are clinically confirmatory (Figure 9.18C).

Investigations to Consider Ophthalmic and echocardiographic evaluation are indicated in MS. Radiology is necessary if Stickler is considered likely—you will see coronal clefts and flared metaphyses in early life. Lysyl hydroxylase assay on fibroblasts for EDS type VI is usually diagnostic, being functionally absent. Serum tenascin X assay is indicated for any clinically suspected cases of EDS.

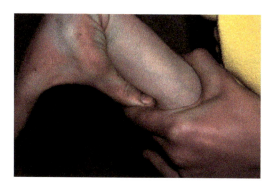

Figure 11.7A Typical hypermobility of the thumb is demonstrated in a patient with type III Ehlers-Danlos syndrome.

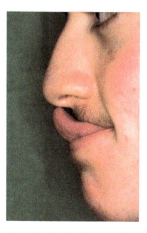

Figure 11.7B Gorlin sign, the ability to touch the nasal tip with the tongue, is a feature of many cases of Ehlers-Danlos syndrome but is seen in fewer than 10% of the non–Ehlers-Danlos population.

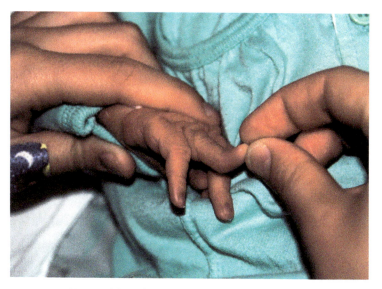

Figure 11.7C Hypermobility of the distal interphalangeal joint is demonstrated in this baby with Ehlers-Danlos syndrome type II. Note the excess skin over the hands, manifesting as additional skin wrinkling over the fifth finger.

11.8 Small or Absent Patella

Recognizing the Sign Clinically, the clue to patellar absence or hypoplasia is of a flat anterior aspect to the knee, accentuated on flexion. The patella is not palpable and is not seen radiologically. A pitfall for the unwary is that in young children patellar ossification may be delayed until as late as age 6 years in the normal population.

Establishing a Differential Diagnosis Single gene diseases may be flagged by the family history. In particular, **nail-patella syndrome** (NPS), being autosomal dominant, may be recognized in other family members. A family history of renal failure in one or more individuals, typically becoming symptomatic in early adulthood, in combination with clinical signs of nail malformation, especially in the thumbs and index fingers, and triangular shape to the lunules are characteristic of the disorder, effectively confirming the diagnosis. The absence of skin creases over the distal interphalangeal joints is a common observation (Figure 12.1). Patellar agenesis is a feature of a more widespread bone dysplasia representing mild **camptomelic dysplasia**, a condition that is usually associated with severe tibial bowing and dimpling and often associated with respiratory compromise and death. However, in attenuated form, survivors may show few clinical features apart from patellar hypoplasia. Radial defects, including absence of the thumbs, in combination with patellar hypoplasia are suggestive of a group of molecularly related disorders represented by **Rothmund-Thompson syndrome**. Short stature, skin mottling, telangiectasia, and craniosynostosis are other features of this variable group of conditions, which are autosomal recessively inherited. A less disparate phenotype is that of **Meier-Gorlin syndrome**, in which autosomal recessive disorder short stature is associated with hypoplastic patellae. The best guide to the diagnosis is the small ears, which are unmistakable. In a child with unexplained developmental delay, always examine for absent patellae, the identification of which is very likely to signify **mosaic trisomy 8**. The diagnosis may be confirmed clinically by checking for the deep plantar creases (Figure 10.6). If associated with contractures of the knees and/or severe talipes, do bear in mind the possibility of **genitopatellar syndrome**, in which the presence of scrotal hypoplasia, cryptorchidism, and clitoromegaly are to be anticipated on examination and severe developmental delay likely.

Investigations to Consider Renal biochemistry and urinary albumin-to-creatinine ratio annually are recommended for NPS patients as a screen for incipient renal disease. Mutation of *LMX1B* confirms the diagnosis. Skeletal radiology will establish abnormal ischiopubic ossification in surviving camptomelic dysplasia cases. *RECQL4* mutations are established in Rothmund-Thompson syndrome and related phenotypes. Mosaic trisomy 8 generally requires fibroblast culture to establish the cytogenetic abnormality.

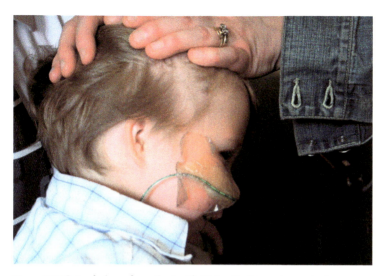

Figure 11.8 Lateral view of a patient with Meier-Gorlin syndrome to demonstrate the typical microtia that identifies the condition from a host of other short stature disorders.

11.9 Pseudoarthrosis

Recognizing the Sign Most typically a feature of tibial fracture, pseudoarthrosis refers to the nonunion of a long bone following fracture resulting, usually, in a permanent localized area of discontinuity in the shaft of the bone. Although congenital presentation is known, the more usual history is of progressive bowing of the limb in the first year of life and spontaneous fracture on attempted weight bearing, there being subsequent nonunion of the fracture.

Establishing a Differential Diagnosis Establish whether the long bones are normal elsewhere with respect to length and absence of deformation, or bowing. The major diagnostic concern is for **Neurofibromatosis type 1** (NF1). While characteristic skin changes of multiple café-au-lait patches, axillary and groin freckling, and palpable neurofibroma are typical in the older child, readily facilitating diagnosis, the disorder is easily overlooked when presentation predates the onset of cutaneous clues. Obviously, parental examination for signs of this autosomal dominant condition is important in any child presenting with pseudoarthrosis. In evaluating such a case, it is useful to be aware that the absence of Lisch nodules—benign hamartomas of the iris typically seen in NF1—on iris examination does not reduce the likelihood of NF1, since these are rarely observed in children under the age of 5 years. Since many cases of NF1 arise as de novo mutations, serial examination for emerging café-au-lait patches is appropriate in a child presenting with a pseudoarthrosis, as is parental history and examination. Potential for diagnostic confusion exists in that **McCune-Albright syndrome** also presents cutaneous pigmentary abnormalities and cystic lesions of bones, occasionally associated with fracture. The pigmentary abnormalities, though said to mimic café-au-lait patches, are usually irregular in outline, in contrast with the typically smooth outline of a café-au-lait patch in NF1 (Figure 12.8). The presence of endocrine abnormalities, perhaps presenting clinically with precocious puberty or hyperthyroidism, is a good basis for differentiation from NF1. Fibrous dysplasia of bone, mimicking pseudoarthrosis and sometimes associated with bowing, is well described in **Mulibrey Nanism**, an autosomal recessive disorder associated with growth failure and which clinically resembles Silver-Russell syndrome.

Investigations to Consider Optic nerve evaluation for optic glioma is indicated in NF1, and serial blood pressure measurement is recommended in view of associated renal artery stenosis and pheochromocytoma. Mutation of *GNAS1* is diagnostic of McCune-Albright, and thyroid function tests are important considerations in management. Skeletal radiology shows slender long bones with a narrow medullary channel and occasionally fibrous dysplasia of the fibula in Mulibrey Nanism. Echocardiography or magnetic resonance imaging is advised for possible constrictive pericarditis.

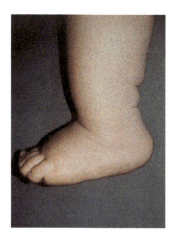

Figure 11.9A A very typical anterior deformity of the lower limb is shown in a child with neurofibromatosis type 1–related pseudoarthrosis. (Courtesy of Dr. Susan Huson.)

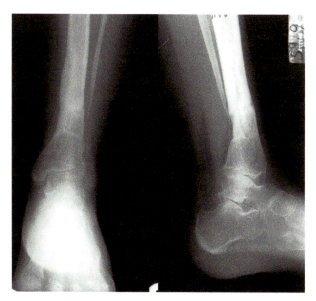

Figure 11.9B Radiologic appearance of neurofibromatosis type 1–related pseudoarthrosis is shown in a different case. (Courtesy of Dr. J. Kelleher.)

11.10 Madelung Deformity

Recognizing the Sign Madelung deformity is a clinical sign that emerges as a child grows. It generally takes 5 or 6 years for the feature to become identifiable. Bony growth is disproportionate in the forearm, the distal end of the ulna becoming progressively dorsally dislocated. Clinically, the forearm adopts a very recognizable appearance, sometimes referred to as "dinner-fork" configuration, there being a dip between the distal end of the ulna and the wrist. Generally, there is associated mesomelia (middle segment of the limb, hence forearm and tibia + fibula) and short stature. There may be some restriction of elbow extension. Radiologically, the radius is short with respect to the ulna and usually bowed, and the distal radial epiphysis shows a sloping outline.

Establishing a Differential Diagnosis This is the clinical signature par excellence of **Leri-Weill syndrome**. The affected child usually presents to the pediatric clinic with short stature. A background history of short stature may be noted in the family, and parental examination may establish similar forearm and wrist deformations. Intelligence and other developmental parameters are normal. The condition is described as autosomal dominant, affecting both male and female patients, although the gene is on the short arm of the X chromosome, in the pseudoautosomal region, thus explaining this apparent deviation from classical genetic principles of inheritance. The main differential diagnosis is from patients with **Turner syndrome** and others with localized deletions of the Xp22 chromosomal region. Both such patient groups are short and more likely to show Madelung deformity due to absence of the pseudoautosomal region of the X chromosome.

Investigations to Consider Skeletal radiology confirms the typical appearance of the radius and ulna, often with associated shortening of the tibia and, even more, of the fibula. Karyotype is useful, not only for the identification of Turner syndrome, but also because several cases with deletion of Xp22-ter have been recorded with Madelung deformity. Submicroscopic deletions and mutations of the *SHOX* gene on Xp22 have been demonstrated in several affected families.

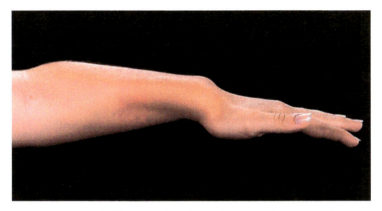

Figure 11.10A A typical instance of Madelung forearm is shown. Note the "dinner-fork" configuration of the wrist.

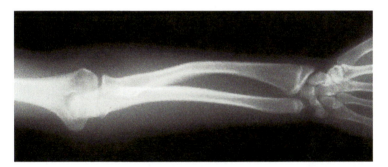

Figure 11.10B The radiology confirms the radial bowing and the distal radial epiphysis presents a sloping appearance. (Courtesy of Dr. Debbie Shears.)

Chapter 12 **The Nails, Hair, and Skin**

12.1 Absent or Hypoplastic Nails

Recognizing the Sign Absent nails are simply a matter of observation, but hypoplastic nails are a subjective judgment. Complete absence of the nails is very uncommon. If nail hypoplasia is signifying an underlying syndromic diagnosis, the nail abnormality will be readily identifiable. Small nails are usually deeply embedded in the tissue surrounding them, the term "deep set" being apt.

Establishing a Differential Diagnosis In a neonate, consider teratogenic causes and in particular exposure to **alcohol** or **phenytoin** during pregnancy. In both disorders parallel effects would be anticipated in the feet, and the absence of such clinical findings should call for caution in attributing the syndrome. Family history can offer clues—in particular, dominant **ectodermal dysplasia** with sparse growth of fine hair, dystrophic nails, and abnormalities of dentition may explain the clinical findings. The possibility of a diaphragmatic hernia in a neonate should prompt assessment for **Fryns syndrome**, one of the cardinal features of which is small nails. Coarse facial features, increased birth weight above the norm, and corneal clouding are important pointers toward this autosomal recessive condition. Deep-set nails are a cardinal feature of **Ellis-van Creveld (E-vC) syndrome** and should prompt evaluation for this possible diagnosis. Evidence of postaxial polydactyly, possibly in the form of a tiny irregularity on the ulnar margin of the fifth finger; accessory frenula and natal teeth; narrow chest; and low birth length are all suggestive of the disorder. If suspected, then cardiac evaluation is important, the most common lesion being an atrial septal defect (ASD). Nail dysplasia concentrated on the radial side of the hand, frequently with normal nails on fingers 3 to 5, is suggestive of **nail-patella syndrome** (NPS). Look for the characteristic triangular shape to the lunules, loss of creases over the distal interphalangeal (DIP) joints of the fingers, and absent, impalpable, or easily dislocated patella. There is a significant risk (>10%) of developing kidney disease. Nail hypoplasia associated with neonatal hypotonia and difficulty in establishing feeding is a typical presentation of **deafness-onycho-osteodystrophy retardation (DOOR) syndrome**. Neonatal seizures complicate many cases of this autosomal recessive condition. Recognizing the importance of the nail hypoplasia as the key to the diagnosis is the seminal diagnostic maneuver.

Investigations to Consider Echocardiography is indicated in E-vC syndrome, in addition to radiology for narrow thorax and hypoplastic iliac wings. The risk of renal disease in NPS requires annual screening by blood pressure and urine analysis. Urine albumin-to-creatinine ratio is the recommended assay. Mutation of the *LMX1B* gene confirms the diagnosis, if there is clinical doubt. Brainstem auditory-evoked responses show no response to high-intensity stimulation in DOOR syndrome.

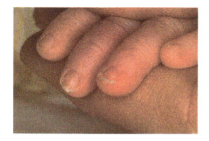

Figure 12.1A Shown are nails that are small and deep set. The nails themselves look normal, but observe how small they are relative to the distance from the distal interphalangeal joint crease.

A

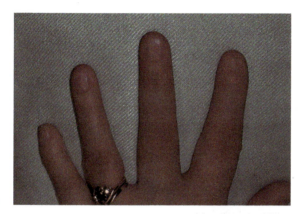

B

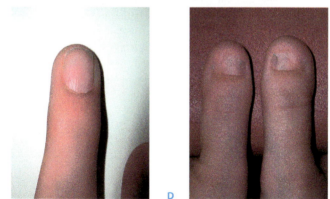

C

D

Figure 12.1B–D Diagnostically valuable signs in the hand of patients with nail-patella syndrome are demonstrated. Note the normal nails on fingers 3 to 5 but the small index finger nail. The triangular outline of the lunules in fingers 3 to 5 is also well demonstrated. Distal interphalangeal joint creases are also absent, as is expected. The dysplastic thumb nails are also typical, the thumbs and index fingers characteristically showing more severe degrees of nail dysplasia. (Courtesy of Prof. Ian Young and Dr. Ernie Bongers.)

12.2 "Tale of a Nail" Sign

Recognizing the Sign A hooked nail of the fifth finger, specifically, of unusual shape due to its adherence to a hypoplastic distal phalanx of the finger comprises the "tale of a nail" sign. Minor variations of this arise, sometimes extending to small volar nails on the palmar surface of the fifth finger. The muscle pulp of the distal fifth finger is often significantly and noticeably reduced.

Establishing a Differential Diagnosis In almost all cases, this rare sign is signifying **deletion of chromosome 4q34**. Very few cases are described, but swallowing difficulties, frequently complicated by aspiration, are especially common among affected individuals. Associated congenital heart disease is also well recognized. It is worth obtaining a family history, since the condition, in less florid form, can be associated with essentially normal development and parent-to-child transmission is known, the parent having been spared the aspiration and associated respiratory difficulties that may bedevil the child. As with any chromosomal deletion syndrome, the clinical features are variable, but developmental delay is frequent among those who are recognized and survive the aspiration-related risks. It is likely that many pediatric cases of recurrent aspiration have this little-known condition.

Investigations to Consider The basic karyotype is often reported as normal. Specific direction of cytogenetic attention may reveal a submicroscopic deletion of the 4q34 region on higher band scrutiny, but occasionally molecular cytogenetics, perhaps by way of subtelomeric fluorescent in situ hybridization (FISH) or array hybridization may have to be resorted to, if the deletion is to be revealed.

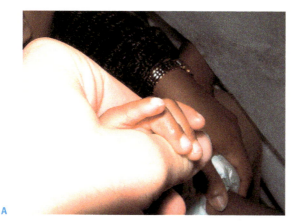

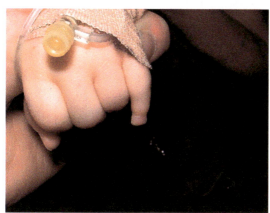

Figure 12.2A and B The nails of two children with 4q34 deletions are shown. Note the variation in the clinical sign and the demonstration of the hypoplasia of the muscle pulp on the palmar surface of the digit.

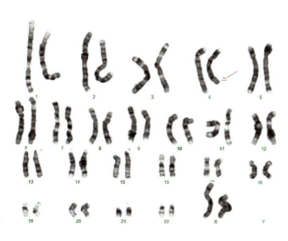

Figure 12.2C The minute deletion of chromosome 4q34 is shown on the karyotype; the original report, at lower levels of investigation, was reported as normal.

12.3 Longitudinal Splitting of the Nails

Recognizing the Sign Most characteristic of the thumb but also seen in other digits, including the feet, longitudinal ridges, which are both visible and palpable, traverse the length of the nail and the patient or parent will report that the nail routinely breaks at this fault line. In the neonatal period, it is often easier to feel this sign than to see it.

Establishing a Differential Diagnosis Few signs are pathognomonic, but the recognition of this sign in a female patient is strongly suggestive of **craniofrontonasal dysplasia** (CFND). In florid form, the patient will present with hypertelorism and plagiocephaly at birth and a diagnosis of craniosynostosis will be reached without specifying a particular syndrome. The recognition of this clinical sign identifies the underlying condition but is also prognostically important, CFND being generally associated with a normal developmental outcome, not the universal experience in other forms of craniosynostosis. Diagnostic and prognostic confusion can be exponentially increased in the unrecognized case by the identification on imaging of an absent corpus callosum, usually a poor prognostic indicator in developmental terms but a normal finding in many patients with CFND. Other clinical features that, if present, support this likely diagnosis are a bifid nasal tip, widow's peak hair line, and wiry texture to the hair in the older patient. Breast asymmetry and sloping shoulders, with enhanced shoulder joint hypermobility, mimicking cleidocranial dysostosis, are also well recognized within the CFND clinical spectrum. Almost all cases described are female, there being few convincing male cases.

Investigations to Consider Skull x-rays may be indicated to establish whether there is synostosis of the coronal or other sutures. Mutation analysis of the *EFNB1* gene confirms if there is a clinical doubt.

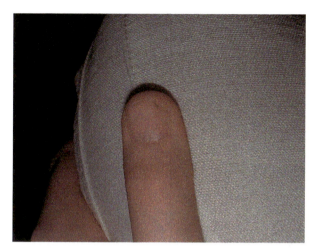

Figure 12.3A A typical instance of longitudinal splitting of a thumb nail is demonstrated in an adult patient with craniofrontonasal dysplasia.

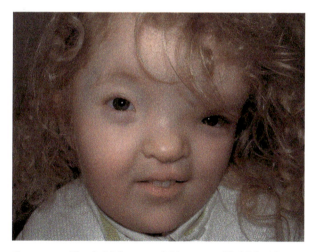

Figure 12.3B The facial features of this 3-year-old child with craniofrontonasal dysplasia are unlikely to be confused with any other syndrome. Note the hypertelorism and bifid nasal tip. The corpus callosum is absent but development is normal.

12.4 Short Nails

Recognizing the Sign There is not a clear-cut distinction between short nails and small nails, which will obviously overlap somewhat with nails described as dysplastic. However, what the clinician notes is that the nails are short in the longitudinal axis. Obviously this is to be anticipated in cases of brachydactyly (see 9.7), where the nail shortening reflects a generalized shortness of the phalanges. In contrast with dysplastic nails, the nail growth and strength are normal.

Establishing a Differential Diagnosis Though rare, **cartilage-hair hypoplasia (CHH) syndrome** is an important condition to establish in infancy because of the associated susceptibility to varicella. Short stature is usually apparent at birth or shortly afterward, but the head circumference is normal. Scalp hair is sparse and fine, though this sign tends to be more valuable in the postneonatal period. Recurrent infections or low white cells can offer additional clues to the diagnosis. In all cases seen by the author, short nails were a valuable clinical sign noted on the first examination, predating the diagnosis and signaling appropriate investigations. Short nails are common in **Williams syndrome**, though it is the typical facial features of anteverted nostrils with a long philtrum and progressive thickening of the lips that are more likely to betray this diagnosis to a clinician. However, in a child with a murmur, especially if related to supravalvular aortic stenosis or pulmonary stenosis, the recognition of short nails should accentuate the case for specific genetic investigation of Williams syndrome. Progressive loss of energy in a clinically normal child should always prompt investigation of renal biochemistry. This is even more appropriate in the context of short nails, which may the only clinically identifiable abnormality in **Mainzer-Saldino syndrome**. Chronic renal failure due to nephronophthisis is the usual presentation, but a pigmentary retinopathy should be sought, as it foretells the predestined eventual tunnel vision. In view of the occasional association with anatomic malformations of the cerebellum, such as Dandy-Walker malformation, it is worth seeking a history of delayed motor milestones and examining clinically for ataxia.

Investigations to Consider Differential white cell count in CHH syndrome may disclose a neutropenia or lymphopenia. Skeletal radiology shows metaphyseal dysplasia, most characteristically at the lower end of the femora. FISH of *ELN* on chromosome 7 confirms the localized deletion typical of Williams syndrome. Urinary concentration defects usually predate abnormal urea and creatinine in Mainzer-Saldino syndrome, so look for polyuria, nonspecific aminoaciduria, and glycosuria.

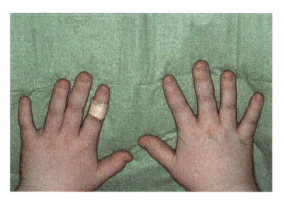

Figure 12.4 The very short nails in this 9-year-old girl presenting with advanced renal failure and a creatinine level of 1,400 μm/L were the clinical clues to the underlying diagnosis of Mainzer-Saldino syndrome. Retinal examination confirmed the expected pigmentary retinopathy.

12.5 Temporal Balding

Recognizing the Sign Although the hair grows well elsewhere without localized areas of alopecia, there is poor growth of hair on the temporal regions, which have a high anterior hairline in consequence.

Establishing a Differential Diagnosis Sparse temporal hair growth is one of the classical clinical hallmarks of **Pallister-Killian syndrome**. This condition is caused by tetrasomy of chromosome 12p, but the abnormal chromosome finding rarely manifests on routine chromosomal analysis. Hence, clinical recognition and directed karyotypic investigation are critical if the diagnosis is to be established. Temporal balding is a cornerstone of that clinical recognition process (Figure 3.5C). Affected children will present with severe developmental delay and do not usually acquire speech. The family history is noncontributory. The face tends to be slightly coarse, becoming more so with age, and the cheeks can assume a somewhat sagging appearance. Accessory nipples are frequent and lend support to the likely diagnosis. The condition may present prenatally with polyhydramnios or neonatally with diaphragmatic hernia. A much better developmental prognosis attends **tricho-rhino-phalangeal (TRP) syndrome**, in which autosomal dominant condition evaluation of the parents may signal the diagnosis. In addition to sparse wispy hair, notably deficient at the temples, the nose is often slightly unusual with a prominent tip and relative deficiency of the ala nasi (Figure 2.4). Examination of the fingers is valuable because of a slightly crooked appearance, not invariably present but diagnostically valuable if noted, due to deviation at the proximal interphalangeal joints. Temporal balding and a prominent nose of rather pinched appearance are the hallmarks of **Hallermann-Streiff syndrome**. The face is small but the nose striking. In particular, there is noteworthy micrognathia. The eyes appear small and examination almost always reveals cataract. Such hair as there is on the scalp is thin and eyebrows and lashes are likewise sparse. The condition is diagnosed clinically and most cases are intellectually normal.

Investigations to Consider Fibroblast examination for tetrasomy chromosome 12p is the usual means of establishing the diagnosis in Pallister-Killian syndrome. The condition is mosaic and the abnormal isochromosome is not present in all cells. With age, it becomes less likely that the isochromosome will be identified. Hence, repeated analysis can be necessary for confirmation. Hand x-rays in TRP syndrome show short phalanges and cone-shaped epiphyses. A proportion of cases show exostoses, particularly if associated with a microscopically visible deletion at chromosome 8q24.12.

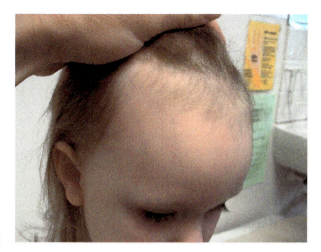

A

B

Figure 12.5A and B Note the large area of temporofrontal region devoid of any hair growth in this 3-year-old girl who had trichorhinophalangeal syndrome. The hands show the typical phalangeal crookedness at the proximal interphalangeal joint. (See also Figures 2.4A and B.)

12.6 Sparse Hair/Alopecia

Recognizing the Sign Subtlety is not required. The hair either does not grow or else is sparse, the scalp being easily visible.

Establishing a Differential Diagnosis Family history may hold the key. Ectodermal dysplasias frequently involve poor hair growth, alopecia, or thin, wiry hair, and several of these syndromes are transmitted from generation to generation. The most common form, **X-linked hypohidrotic ectodermal dysplasia** (Figure 3.15D), is associated with inability to sweat and affected boys often present in infancy with unexplained high fevers. Sparse hair, absent teeth, and deficient eyebrows and eyelashes are good indicators of other affected individuals in the pedigree. Clinical signs are less reliable in carrier females. In the neonatal period, scaling of skin in affected males can lead to confusion with ichthyosis, but the family history and examination offer a ready means of differentiation. An erythematous or seborrheic rash emerging after several months in a child whose skin had previously been normal and alopecia or very sparse hair are the usual harbingers of **biotinidase deficiency**. Often there will have been background concerns about hypotonia and, perhaps, developmental delay. With later presentation the neurologic issues will be more overt and seizures will be recorded. A good clue from the history is to establish whether there have been recurrent fungal infections, to which children with this condition are prone. Neurologic issues again dominate the history in children with **Coffin-Siris syndrome**, severe mental retardation being a consistent finding among these cases. Good clinical pointers to this, apart from the sparse scalp hair, are hypertrichosis over the back and absent fifth fingernails and toenails. The diagnosis is essentially confined to female patients and, though the exact cause is not known, males are rarely diagnosed with this disorder. A history of a cardiac murmur or echocardiographic evidence of interventricular septal thickening and sparse hair growth should pose the question as to whether the child may have **cardiofaciocutaneous (CFC) syndrome**. The skin might be dry, indeed appear ichthyotic, and the liver and spleen enlarged. There is poor hair growth. Often the hair that does grow is curly and the face resembles that of Noonan syndrome, ptosis being common. In the context of a short stature neonate, sparse hair should raise the diagnostic thought of **cartilage–hair-hypoplasia** (CHH), an important diagnosis because of the associated susceptibility to varicella and the immunization implications.

Investigations to Consider Organic aciduria is usually present in biotinidase deficiency. Skeletal radiology shows metaphyseal changes, characteristically most severe at the lower end of the femur in CHH. Mutation analysis of *RMRP* gene confirms.

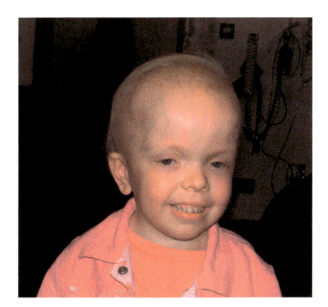

Figure 12.6 The 3-year-old girl pictured here presented with severe eczema in the neonatal period, sparse hair that hardly grew, and a thickened interventricular septum on echocardiography. Unexplained hepatomegaly led to a suggestion that liver biopsy was necessary. However, the recognition of cardio-facio-cutaneous syndrome offered a unifying diagnosis for all these features.

12.7 Poliosis

Recognizing the Sign Loss of melanin production in hair follicles is normal from the fourth decade of life resulting in greying. Poliosis refers to premature greying in childhood or early adulthood.

Establishing a Differential Diagnosis As an aid to diagnosis, poliosis is valuable in **Waardenburg syndrome** (WS), in which deafness, segregating in autosomal dominant manner, should be carefully sought. Several different phenotypes of WS are described, but the important distinction clinically is to establish whether dystopia canthorum is present. This refers to lateral displacement of the inner canthi of the eyes, conferring an impression of hypertelorism on inspection of the face. Examine for slight medial fusion of the eyelids, consequent reduction in the sclera visible medially and lateral displacement of the lacrimal punctum toward the iris. Dystopia canthorum is the hallmark of WS type I, which is genetically distinct from type II, characterized by the absence of this finding. Other diagnostically useful signs to observe are pigment abnormalities, such as heterochromia iridum and hypopigmented skin patches, as well as synophrys, all of which are more common in WS type I–affected individuals and lend diagnostic support. Useful tricks in establishing the diagnosis are to question adult members of the family as to whether they employ hair dyes and to examine the eyelashes, which may be the sole site of poliosis in some affected individuals. The main scope for clinical error is confusion with **piebaldism** (12.11). Patients affected by **Williams syndrome** are unlikely to present with poliosis in the early childhood period, the cardiac murmur, hypercalcemia, and constipation being more likely features to bring them to attention. However, cases missed in childhood who present in adolescence for diagnosis of unexplained developmental delay are usually recognizable by their somewhat coarse facial features and frequent poliosis. **Ataxia telangiectasia** cases generally develop normally until walking, at which time ataxia becomes apparent. Scleral telangiectasia, a history of sun sensitivity, and poliosis should be sought if this diagnosis is being considered.

Investigations to Consider Good audiologic profiling is obviously important if WS is being considered and may need to be extended to other family members. Mutation of *PAX3* gene is confirmatory of type I, mutation of *MITF* being seen in type II. Mutation at other loci, such as *SOX10*, can also present a WS-like picture clinically. If Williams syndrome is suspected, the FISH of *ELN* on chromosome 7q should establish the characteristic deletion. Elevated serum α-fetoprotein is a good screening test for ataxia telangiectasia, and confirmation is established by demonstrating increased chromosome breakage following irradiation of cultured cells.

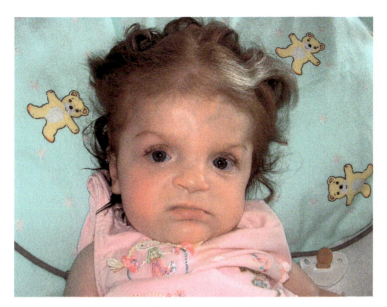

Figure 12.7A A white forelock, the typical form of poliosis in Waardenburg syndrome, is demonstrated in this 1-year-old child with deafness. Note also the clinical impression of hypertelorism occasioned by her dystopia canthorum. In fact, the pupils are not displaced and there is not a true hypertelorism. Although this patient does not show synophrys, the medial flare of the eyebrow, which she does manifest, is also typical of Waardenburg syndrome.

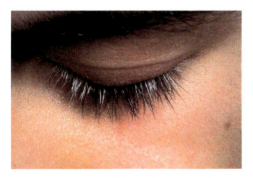

Figure 12.7B Poliosis of the eyelash only is demonstrated, this patient also being deaf.

12.8 Café-au-Lait Patches

Recognizing the Sign These are well-circumscribed brown macules that can arise anywhere on the body. As one or two such pigmentary marks are present in up to 20% of the normal population, the recognition of café-au-lait patches does not, of itself, signify an underlying syndrome but rather begs the question of the clinician as to whether there may be an associated syndrome. An adequate clinical examination needs to address this possibility.

Establishing a Differential Diagnosis The primary condition associated with this clinical finding is **neurofibromatosis type 1** (NF1). A positive background family history and multiple café-au-lait patches in a child secure the diagnosis in clear-cut instances. However, de novo cases or the unavailability of a family history requires adherence to diagnostic criteria. Café-au-lait patches should exceed 0.5 cm in prepubertal individuals to be considered significant. Other cutaneous stigmata to seek out are axillary or groin freckling, usually apparent by the age of 5 years; dermal neurofibromata, which tend to be a feature of late childhood and early adulthood; and plexiform neurofibromata. Ophthalmic evaluation should establish whether there is evidence of optic glioma and should also include slit lamp examination for Lisch nodules, the presence of which further contributes to establishing the diagnosis. Both renal artery stenosis and pheochromocytoma are associated with NF1, and blood pressure evaluation forms an important element of clinical examination. Likewise, spinal assessment for scoliosis is recommended in view of the aggressive nature of scoliosis in NF1 patients. **McCune-Albright syndrome** is characterized by large café-au-lait skin marks that usually have an irregular (coast of Maine) outline and are generally unilateral, respecting the midline. Clinical evidence of precocious puberty should be sought as well as radiologic confirmation of polyostotic fibrous dysplasia. Café-au-lait patches in a patient with short stature should alert the clinician to possible **Russell-Silver syndrome**, about 25% of whom show this feature. Examination for signs of asymmetry and evaluation of the history for low birth weight and characteristically fussy eating may add to the evidence for this diagnosis. Pancytopenia is the ultimate fate of children with **Fanconi syndrome,** but recognition of this autosomal recessive condition prior to hematologic crisis is sometimes possible. Café-au-lait patches, especially if associated with thumb or radial hypoplasia, may be the essential clues.

Investigations to Consider Skeletal radiology is indicated to demonstrate polyostotic lesions in McCune-Albright syndrome, in which evaluation of thyroid function is recommended. Cytogenetic analysis is occasionally warranted, as ring chromosomes can present clinically with café-au-lait patches, almost inevitably associated with developmental delay. Diepoxybutane challenge to chromosomes is the diagnostic test for Fanconi syndrome.

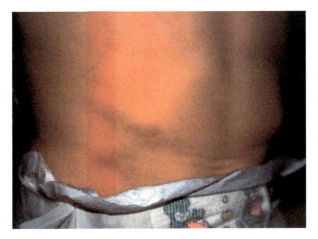

Figure 12.8A Several café-au-lait patches are seen on the abdomen in this patient with neurofibromatosis type 1. Note the oval shape and smooth margin of the pigmented regions.

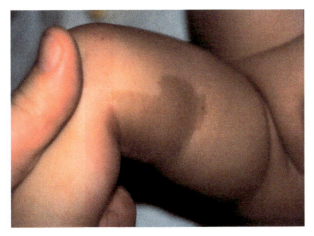

Figure 12.8B The large café-au-lait patch shown in this child, offspring of consanguineous parents, was the clinical feature that facilitated the early diagnosis of the autosomal recessive condition Fanconi anemia.

12.9 Acanthosis Nigricans

Recognizing the Sign This term describes hyperpigmented regions of skin, of velvety appearance, typically distributed in the neck, axillae, and antecubital and popliteal regions. The accentuation of the skin markings differentiates this feature from mere hyperpigmentation.

Establishing a Differential Diagnosis Nowadays, the most common cause of acanthosis nigricans is obesity and, even in the presence of normal nutritional status, most instances of acanthosis nigricans are without syndromic association. However, acanthosis nigricans is an important diagnostic feature in some syndromes. Specifically, **leprechaunism** is associated with this finding. Intrauterine growth retardation, facial hirsutism, and enlarged breasts and genitalia are the usual features of this disorder. A prominent facial feature is lip thickening, and intraoral examination usually reveals gum hypertrophy. Insulin receptor gene mutations underlie leprechaunism, and insulin resistance in any form is associated with this clinical sign. **Lipodystrophy**, whether total or partial, is generally associated with insulin resistance and acanthosis nigricans. The clinical hallmark of lipodystrophy in childhood is the apparent muscularity of the subject, occasioned by the absence of subcutaneous fat. Hepatomegaly, early-onset diabetes mellitus, and hypertrophic cardiomyopathy are all consistent with the diagnosis. Acanthosis nigricans is well described in **Costello syndrome**, in which the typical history of neonatal feeding difficulty, followed by a progressive facial coarsening in the second year of life, prompts the diagnosis on looking at sequential photographs of the child. Excess skin of the hands, mimicking an oversized glove, is a very good clue to this diagnosis, in which cardiomyopathy and increased risk of malignancy is well documented. Absence of the characteristic nasal papillomata is not a bar to diagnosis, as these do not appear until the age of 5 or 6 years (Figure 2.8B). In a child with a clinical and radiologic diagnosis of achondroplasia, the emergence of acanthosis nigricans signifies the more severe form, known as **SADDAN syndrome** (severe achondroplasia, developmental delay, and acanthosis nigricans). Mutation of the *FGFR3* gene causes SADDAN syndrome, but other phenotypes of *FGFR3* mutation are also associated with acanthosis nigricans, specifically a mild form of **Crouzon syndrome** of craniosynostosis.

Investigations to Consider Hyperinsulinemia is characteristic of both leprechaunism and lipodystrophy. Raised lipid levels should be sought in lipodystrophy. Leprechaunism may be confirmed by *INSR* mutation analysis. Costello syndrome is diagnosed clinically, but molecular confirmation by *HRAS* gene on chromosome 11p is available. Like achondroplasia, SADDAN syndrome reflects mutation at the *FGFR3* locus, all reported cases of the latter sharing the A1949T mutation. Mutations elsewhere at this locus cause Crouzon syndrome associated with acanthosis nigricans.

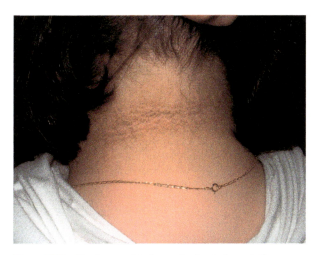

Figure 12.9A Obesity-associated acanthosis nigricans is demonstrated in this overweight 10-year-old girl.

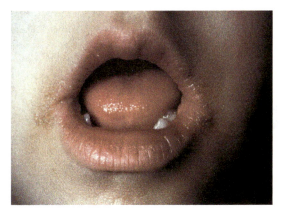

Figure 12.9B Mild perioral acanthosis nigricans in a child who presented with unusual skull shape secondary to craniosynostosis facilitates the diagnosis as a function of *FGFR3* mutation.

12.10 Diffuse Hypopigmented Streaky Lesions

Recognizing the Sign The striking aspect of this sign is the pigmentary disturbance, with linear streaks of hypopigmented regions seen over the limbs and whorls of hypopigmentation seen over the trunk. Skin texture may be slightly more rough or dry over the affected region and, in subtle cases in whom the pigmentary disturbance is not readily identifiable, it is the textural skin differences that may draw the examiner's attention. In such instances, examination with a Wood's lamp in a darkened room is required to reveal the hypopigmentation. Although often present at birth or noted shortly thereafter, hypomelanosis may develop up to the age of 1 year.

Establishing a Differential Diagnosis This is the cardinal clinical sign of **genetic mosaicism** and is most commonly encountered in cases of unexplained developmental delay. Typically, blood karyotype will be normal but fibroblast karyotype may reveal the mosaicism. Other clinical features, such as micrognathia, syndactyly of the fingers, and obesity of adolescent onset, are likely to be associated with the mosaic phenotype. Obesity is particularly noted in patients mosaic for diploid/triploid mosaicism (46XX/69XXX). Most commonly, the mosaicism is chromosomal, there being two discernible and distinct cell lines demonstrable on fibroblast culture, though rarely on lymphoblast culture. However, hypomelanosis is also described in mosaicism for single gene disorders, most notably in heterozygote female carriers of the X-linked condition **Menkes disease**.

Investigations to Consider Karyotype, especially on fibroblasts, is indicated. It should be noted that repeated normal karyotypes have been recorded in some affected individuals. As patients get older, it appears that the likelihood of positive findings on karyotype become reduced, presumably due to selective loss of the abnormal chromosomal cell line in skin cells. Keratinocyte culture is reputed to have a higher yield in terms of identifying abnormal karyotypes among patients with this clinical phenomenon but is not available in most centers.

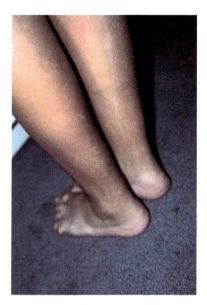

Figure 12.10A Typical hypopigmented linear streaky lesions are seen on the back of the calves in this teenage girl who presented with unexplained developmental delay and seizures. The lesions could be followed upward onto the buttocks and were also visible on the back.

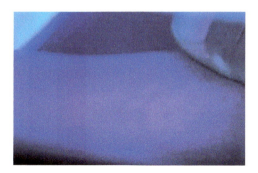

Figure 12.10B This photograph shows subclinical hypopigmentation, identified under Wood's light, in a patient whose presentation was with severe micrognathia, requiring prolonged tracheostomy, and developmental delay of moderate degree. This is the same patient as shown in Figure 2.10.

12.11   Piebaldism

Recognizing the Sign   Local areas of skin hypopigmentation are present from birth, affecting any region of the body. In equine parlance, a "piebald" refers to a horse of two different colors, typically a blotchy combination of black and white.

Establishing a Differential Diagnosis   Blotchy hypopigmentation is typical of autosomal dominant **familial piebaldism**, which is usually readily diagnosable by reference to family history and observation or clinical examination of immediate relatives of the index case. In contrast to **vitiligo**, the hypopigmented regions of piebaldism are present from birth, vitiligo being an acquired form of hypopigmentation. Apart from the cutaneous hypopigmentation, patients with piebaldism almost invariably have a central poliosis. The main differential diagnosis is of **Waardenburg syndrome**, in which patients have poliosis, often with associated dystopia canthorum and deafness, as well as hypopigmented skin regions (Figure 12.7). Since deafness is an occasional but inconstant finding in piebaldism, confident clinical distinction between the two diagnoses may not always be easy. However, in general, the hypopigmentation of pure piebaldism is more noteworthy than that seen in most cases of Waardenburg syndrome. Additional clinical signs in Waardenburg syndrome of heterochromia iridum or brilliant blue eyes with hypoplastic stroma can also assist in differentiation. Hypopigmented skin lesions, occasionally associated with poliosis, are a rare form of clinical presentation of **Fanconi anemia** predating the characteristic pancytopenia by several years but offering an opportunity to the clinically aware of recognizing this autosomal recessive condition in a presymptomatic stage. Sometimes careful examination of the hands may establish mild degrees of thumb hypoplasia, which further lends weight to this possible diagnosis.

Investigations to Consider   The diagnosis is generally clinical. Mutation analysis is possible in familial piebaldism, the relevant genes being *KIT* and *SNAI2*. Karyotype with diepoxybutane challenge is warranted if Fanconi anemia is suspected.

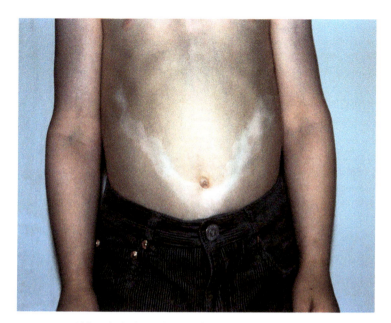

Figure 12.11 Although the hypopigmented regions so dramatically demonstrated in this patient from a pedigree segregating piebaldism as an autosomal dominant trait are symmetric, this need not necessarily be the case in all affected individuals.

12.12 Cutis Marmorata

Recognizing the Sign This is a vascular phenomenon, present at birth and which often fades with time, becoming less noticeable. Essentially, the skin has a "marbled" appearance consequent on a reticular vascular pattern. The mottling of the skin can be exacerbated by changes in temperature or by emotion, so that direct questioning of parents as to the effect of bathing or of crying on the skin pigmentation can be a useful aspect of history taking.

Establishing a Differential Diagnosis The skin marbling appearance may be localized or general and, in the course of assessment, be alive to the possibility of associated limb atrophy or hypertrophy conferring limb asymmetry. While localized limb atrophy associated with cutis marmorata is well established as an isolated and nonsyndromic phenomenon, the finding of limb asymmetry also raises the possibility of **macrocephaly-cutis marmorata-telangiectasia congenita (MCTC) syndrome.** In this distinct overgrowth syndrome, macrocephaly and cutis marmorata are associated with limb asymmetry, occasional polydactyly, a very typical 2/3 syndactyly of the toes, and a degree of developmental delay. The very characteristic facial feature is of a hemangioma on the philtrum. A similar but clinically distinct disorder is **Klippel-Trenaunay-Weber syndrome** (KTW), in which limb asymmetry is associated with macular vascular nevi and intelligence and developmental parameters are normal. The philtral hemangioma and 2/3 toe syndactyly of MCTC syndrome are lacking on examination in K-T-W cases. Cutis marmorata in the distribution of the trigeminal branch of the fifth cranial nerve is well described in association with glaucoma and, as such, overlaps clinically with **Sturge-Weber syndrome** (S-WS), the typical trigeminal lesion of which is a hemangioma. In view of this overlap, the possibility of associated meningeal angiomata, seizures, and neurologic deficit should be borne in mind if the distribution of the skin mottling is confined to this region. Neonatal hypotonia, difficulty in establishing feeding, the impression of macroglossia, and cutis marmorata should alert the clinician to the possibility of **Down syndrome,** and these same clinical features may also betoken **congenital hypothyroidism.** Constipation is a frequent complaint in both these situations.

Investigations to Consider Karyotype is indicated if Down syndrome is clinically suspected. Neonatal screening will establish congenital hypothyroidism in most instances. Skull radiographs are warranted if Sturge-Weber is suspected. The distribution of the vascular pattern often shows "tram line" calcification, which may be identified in the cortex or in the angiomatous vessels.

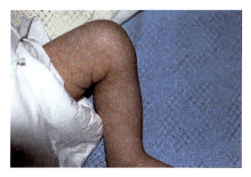

Figure 12.12A The characteristic marbled appearance of cutis marmorata of no syndromic significance is demonstrated in this neonate.

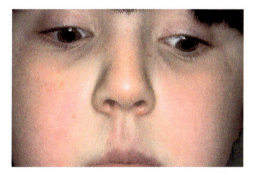

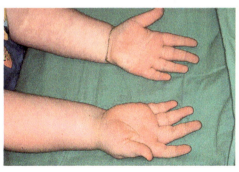

Figure 12.12B and C This photograph shows a 5-year-old girl who presented with developmental delay and limb asymmetry. Note the faded but still discernible triangular-shaped hemangioma over the philtrum. Observe also the prominent vascular marking of the hands and the left forearm especially. The diagnosis in this child is macrocephaly-cutis marmorata-telangiectasia congenita syndrome.

12.13 Capillary Hemangioma

Recognizing the Sign More colloquially known as "strawberry marks," capillary hemangiomas are soft, red areas of raised skin, of which the related history is frequently of a pale or slightly red localized region of skin at birth, which rapidly grows into the typical elevated strawberry nevus during the first year of life, generally regressing thereafter.

Establishing a Differential Diagnosis Most strawberry marks are devoid of any associated diagnostic implications. Indeed, it is estimated that up to 45% of infants have signs of benign vascular marks of this sort. Concern that the hemangioma may have a more particular significance arises if there is a positive family history or if multiple such lesions are observed. Multiple lesions are usually present from birth and likely to be indicative of **disseminated hemangiomatosis** (DH). Such patients are at risk of visceral hemangiomata developing in the liver, gastrointestinal tract, and respiratory tract, the author being personally familiar with recurrent massive hemoptysis in two affected individuals in which the hemangiomatosis involved the trachea. Both patients had only two or three skin lesions, and these were quite small and had been dismissed as "normal" in the neonatal period. It appears that recognition of DS cases from background "normal" capillary hemangioma requires care and continued surveillance. Thrombocytopenia resulting from an associated Kasabach-Merritt phenomenon is a well-established complication, as is cardiac failure. **Familial forms** are rare and sometimes clinically overlap with a group of genetic disorders that cause familial predisposition to cerebral hemorrhage and retinal hemorrhage, which are transmitted in autosomal dominant mode and associated with specific gene mutations. However, other forms of familial strawberry nevus are devoid of these catastrophic consequences and appear only to segregate cutaneous signs. **Maffucci syndrome** combines the association of hemangioma with enchondromata of the bones, most commonly manifest as bowing clinically of the affected bone. Careful, serial clinical evaluation of the hands, feet, and limbs is required to recognize this condition, with many patients being recognized only subsequent to fracture related to enchondroma.

Investigations to Consider Platelet count and cardiac function need continuous monitoring if Kasabach-Merritt phenomenon arises with consequent thrombocytopenia. Magnetic resonance imaging scanning for individuals at risk of cerebral bleeding is appropriate if the family history suggests one of the dominant forms with this complication.

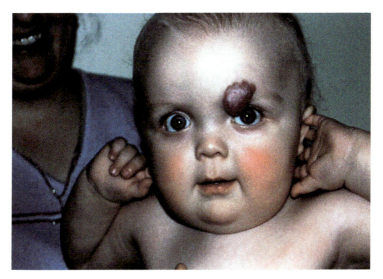

Figure 12.13 A typical capillary hemangioma, which regressed over the next 3 years, is shown in this 11-month-old boy who presented with developmental delay due to a chromosomal disorder. The hemangioma was of no diagnostic significance.

12.14   Telangiectasia

Recognizing the Sign   Prominent blood vessels, of capillary origin, are visible on the skin, conjunctiva, nail beds, and tongue or around the lips. With age, these tend to become more prominent and to increase numerically.

Establishing a Differential Diagnosis   Telangiectasia is almost always significant in the pediatric setting. The interpretation of the sign as a diagnostic indicator will depend on the background history. In a child with normal growth parameters presenting with recurrent epistaxis, the possibility of **hereditary hemorrhagic telangiectasia** (HHT) should be considered. Although skin telangiectasia may not develop until adulthood, being autosomal dominant, parental telangiectasia and/or a history of epistaxis or gastrointestinal bleeding in the family may offer the key to diagnosis. Careful examination of the mucosal surfaces for telangiectasia in the index case may confirm the diagnosis clinically. Be aware of possible major arteriovenous malformations that can result in central nervous system presentations or massive hemoptysis if present in the pulmonary system and for which mechanical embolization may be a treatment option. By contrast, skin telangiectasia in a child whose growth is the cause of concern opens the possibility of **chromosome breakage syndromes** as the underlying cause, all of which conditions have long-term associations with lymphomas and leukemia. A history of prenatal growth deficiency, sun sensitivity, and telangiectasia in a butterfly distribution on the malar region favors **Bloom syndrome**, while growth failure of postnatal onset, coupled with developmental delay and ataxia, is more reminiscent of **ataxia-telangiectasia (AT) syndrome**. Careful neurologic examination may establish evidence of athetosis, dysarthria, or nystagmus, all of which support the diagnosis of AT syndrome. Conjunctival telangiectasia should be sought, as these predate the cutaneous signs that, when established, are typically distributed over the eyelids, malar region, and ears. Sun sensitivity is often the initial diagnostic clue in **Cockayne syndrome**, the typical history being of postnatal growth failure with progressive neurologic concerns, mental retardation, ataxia, weakness, and deafness being common findings. Evaluating early photographs can be valuable, demonstrating a progressive loss of periorbital adipose tissue, the eyes appearing to become more sunken with time. Ophthalmic examination often establishes a diagnostically valuable pigmentary retinopathy. Normal chromosomes characterize **dyskeratosis congenita**, an X-linked condition also resulting in immune compromise and pancytopenia in the second decade and associated with telangiectasia. The presence of dysphagia, leukoplakia, and tear duct blockage all suggest preferment of this latter diagnosis.

Investigations to Consider   Elevated α-fetoprotein is typical in AT syndrome. X irradiation of chromosomes to demonstrate the enhanced breakage under such conditions confirms. Sister chromatid exchange is increased in Bloom syndrome. Ultraviolet irradiation forms the basis of diagnosis in Cockayne syndrome, mRNA synthesis being greatly reduced.

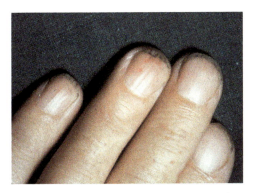

Figure 12.14A Nail telangiectasis is demonstrated in an adult patient with hereditary hemorrhagic telangiectasia syndrome.

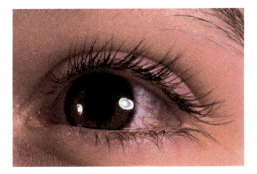

Figure 12.14B Conjunctival telangiectasia demonstrated in a patient with ataxia telangiectasia

12.15 Ichthyosis

Recognizing the Sign This term describes excessively dry, scaly skin reflecting disordered keratinization. Depending on the nature and extent of scaling, quite clinically disparate conditions may be described by ichthyosis.

Establishing a Differential Diagnosis At its most dramatic, ichthyosis is the clinical sign par excellence of **collodion baby syndrome**. The newborn is enmeshed within a shiny membrane, often fissured, which proceeds to exfoliate over the succeeding weeks. Despite the dramatic presentation, a normal neurologic and developmental outcome should be anticipated, and the eventual outlook for the skin is of a mildly dry skin, with normal hair. The condition is autosomal recessive. A family history of dry skin may betray the **autosomal dominant form of ichthyosis**, often associated with atopic dermatitis and asthma. In evaluating male patients referred for nonspecific developmental delay, the identification of dry skin should remind the clinician to inquire as to the history of the delivery. Boys affected with the X-linked recessive condition **steroid sulfatase deficiency** are usually the product of induced labor for prolonged pregnancy, as their carrier mothers produce inadequate estriol and may not labor spontaneously. This condition may be due to localized deletion of the Xp chromosome, and chondrodysplasia punctata, short stature, and Kallmann syndrome may all be observed as part of the related phenotype. However, mutation within the gene results in steroid sulfatase deficiency alone, development being normal and the only clues being the history of delayed onset of labor and ichthyosis. In some cases, the ichthyosiform element of the skin manifestation is quite inapparent, but close inspection may reveal raindrop pigmentation of the skin. The presence of limb shortening or asymmetry is likely to represent **Conradi-Hunnerman syndrome,** an X-linked dominant condition that is rarely compatible with survival in males and therefore is to be suspected clinically in females with ichthyosis. A very characteristic and useful sign is follicular atrophoderma, conferring the appearance of "orange peel" on the skin of the affected individual. Cataracts are another valuable diagnostic sign, as is punctuate calcification of the bones, often a transient finding, for which reason early radiologic evaluation is important if this is suspected.

Investigations to Consider Chondrodysplasia punctata is seen radiologically in both Conradi-Hunnerman and steroid sulfatase deficiency syndromes. Raised 8-dehydrocholesterol is characteristic of Conradi-Hunnerman cases. FISH of Xp22 may establish a deletion in patients with the more extensive steroid sulfatase phenotype, while mutation within the *ARSC* gene should be anticipated in males with the phenotype confined to placental estriol inadequacy and dermatologic signs of ichthyosis. Plasma steroid sulfatase levels are usually unrecordable in both forms of the disorder.

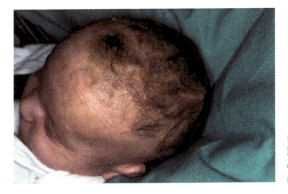

Figure 12.15A Congenital lamellar ichthyosis causing collodion presentation is shown in the recovery phase.

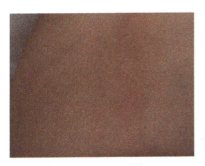

Figure 12.15B A mild degree of ichthyosis is seen in this boy, born by induction of labor after a 43-week gestation, who has steroid sulfatase deficiency, his mother being heterozygous for that condition.

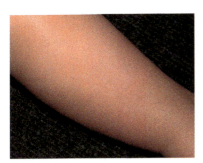

Figure 12.15C Raindrop pigmentation is shown in another boy with an established steroid sulfatase deficiency.

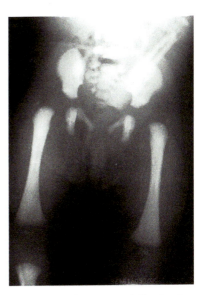

Figure 12.15D Punctuate calcification involving the hip joints is demonstrated in these x-rays from the neonatal period.

12.16 Excess Skin

Recognizing the Sign The clinical impression here will be of a child whose skin is akin to an inappropriately large glove. There may be extra folds of skin in addition to skin wrinkles.

Establishing a Differential Diagnosis Poor feeding in the neonatal period may be the main clue to **Costello syndrome**, in which condition the excess skin is sometimes paralleled by gum hypertrophy and perhaps evidence of cardiomyopathy. By the age of 6 years, the diagnosis becomes apparent with the appearance of the characteristic nasal papillomata (Figure 2.8B). Both **Noonan syndrome** and **cardio-facio-cutaneous syndrome** (CFC) can present with fetal hydrops. However, the more usual presentation is with cardiac concerns, most classically valvular pulmonary stenosis, in the neonatal period. Ptosis, short stature, and prolonged bleeding are characteristic of classic Noonan syndrome cases, sparse curly hair and skin manifestations such as ichthyosis or hemangioma marking the distinction in CFC syndrome. The excess skin is often most apparent over the neck in Noonan syndrome, while CFC cases, like Costello syndrome, frequently show excess skin on the hands. Several children previously described as having **cutis laxa syndrome** more correctly represent examples of Costello syndrome. Similarly, **occipital horn syndrome**, an X-linked condition characterized by easy bruising and scarring with excess joint laxity, can be misdiagnosed as cutis laxa (Figure 6.5). These skeletal features are also typical of the **Ehlers-Danlos syndrome** (EDS) group of disorders. While hyperelasticity of the skin, often associated with scar formation in response to trauma, and joint hypermobility are more reminiscent of types I to III, excess skin is a central element of the diagnosis in type VII. Hip dislocation is especially common in this form, the diagnosis being prompted by the skin fragility and the blue sclera that often attend the condition. Excess skin with associated inverted nipples or unusual distribution of body fat, particularly the observation of fatty pads over the lumbosacral region, are good clues to **carbohydrate-deficient glycoprotein (CDG) syndrome**, in the case of which signs of developmental delay should be sought on examination.

Investigations to Consider Echocardiography has a valuable place in establishing evidence to support the clinical diagnosis of Costello, CFC, and Noonan syndromes. Reduced serum copper and ceruloplasmin is typical of occipital horn syndrome, but the presence of occipital exostoses on skull radiology is the gold-standard investigation (see 6.5). Evidence of a coagulopathy is useful in some forms of CDG syndrome, but the best screening measure for this group of conditions is transferrin isoelectric focusing.

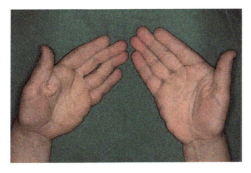

Figure 12.16A The deep palmar creases and general excess of skin are well demonstrated in this teenage patient with Costello syndrome.

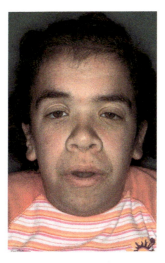

Figure 12.16B The facial features of Costello syndrome in the same patient are shown. Note the facial coarseness, wiry hair, and nasal papillomata. (See also Figure 2.7.)

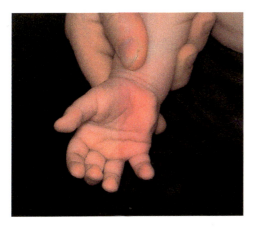

Figure 12.16C Deep palmar creases, excess skin, and fetal finger pads are clearly seen in this hand of a 1-year-old boy with cardiofaciocutaneous syndrome.

It was never envisaged that this should serve as an encyclopedic text on matters dysmorphic and genetic. Rather, this book was conceived as a guide to assist the confident recognition of clinical signs that are often useful in reaching a dysmorphic diagnosis, and thereafter to offer some basic structure to the inexperienced clinician in how to proceed, once secure that he or she had interpreted the clinical signs correctly. The text accompanying each clinical sign is limited by space and, most commonly, this limitation impacts mainly upon the consideration of investigations. Accordingly, readers not habitually accustomed to using genetic resources may benefit from guidance as to where they may seek recourse for further information on specific conditions, journal references, and detailed reports of investigations and their uses in specific clinical settings. Inevitably, such guidance reflects personal practice and preference, the following suggestions being particular favorites to which I turn most commonly but by no means an exhaustive exploration of the many different types of information sources and formats with which a geneticist may have regular cause to interact.

Databases

European Directory of DNA Diagnostic Laboratories (EDDNAL). This is an easy resource for identifying laboratories offering diagnostic DNA testing for specific loci and attendant clinical conditions.

www.eddnal.com

GeneTests. This is a valuable, publicly funded, and therefore free service that allows easy identification of laboratories offering specialized investigations for particular named conditions. It also allows easy access to reviews of particular conditions.

www.geneclinics.org

The Human Gene Mutation Database (HGMD). This is a database containing in excess of 50,000 known mutations in over 2,000 human genes that summarizes and references most of the mutations that have been reported in individual genes and the diseases consequent on mutations therein. It is a useful reference in establishing whether a DNA sequence change has previously been recorded in a pathogenic situation. It is free to academic institutions.

www.hgmd.cf.ac.uk

KnutShell.com. This is a recently launched database online search portal that enables efficient searches of OMIM by symptom or structured list of clinical signs/symptoms. It includes links to GeneTests and indexes of some well established textbooks. Available by individual use-metered or institutional subscription only.

www.knutshell.com

London Medical Databases. This is a constantly updated comprehensive series of linked databases, summarizing all clinical and investigative data on conditions likely to be encountered in a genetics clinic, whether mendelian, chromosomal, or environmental. It is supplemented by a superb library of clinical pictures of each disorder. This is a subscription-only service.

www.lmdatabases.com/contact

OMIM (Online Mendelian Inheritance in Man). This is a constantly updated database, available free of charge, which summarizes clinical and genetic data on mendelian disorders and affords some examples of specific mutations where the locus for a disease has been established.

www.ncbi.nlm.nih.gov/omim/

Radiological Atlas of Malformation Syndromes and Skeletal Dysplasias (REAMS). This is a subscription-only expert system that facilitates searches of known skeletal abnormalities in malformation syndromes and dysplasias by radiologic features, with a view to identifying the most likely conditions to present with these radiologic features.

www.oup.co.uk/ep/cdroms/reams

Books

Aase JM. *Diagnostic dysmorphology.* Published by Plenum Medical Book Co., 1990.

Firth HV, Hurst JA. *Oxford desk reference: Clinical genetics.* Published by Oxford University Press, 2005.

Gardner RJM, Sutherland GR. *Chromosome abnormalities and genetic counselling,* 3rd ed. Published by Oxford University Press, 2004.

Gorlin RJ, Cohen MM Jr, Hennekam RCM. *Syndromes of the head and neck,* 4th ed. Published by Oxford University Press, 2001.

Hall JG, Allanson JE, Gripp KW, Slavotinek AM. *Handbook of physical measurements,* 2nd ed. Published by Oxford University Press, 2006.

Rimoin DL, Connor JM, Pyeritz RE, Korf BR. *Emery and Rimoin's principles and practice of medical genetics,* 4th ed. Published by Churchill Livingstone, 2002.

Spranger JW, Brill P, Poznanski A. *Bone dysplasias: An atlas of genetic disorders of skeletal development,* 2nd ed. Published by Oxford University Press, 2002.

Tabyi H, Lachman RS. *Radiology of syndromes, metabolic disorders and skeletal dysplasias,* 4th ed. Published by Mosby, 1996.

Toriello HV, Reardon W, Gorlin RJ. *Hereditary hearing loss and its syndromes,* 2nd ed. Published by Oxford University Press, 2004.

Traboulsi EI. *Genetic diseases of the eye.* Published by Oxford University Press, 1998.

Index